Freshman Running

A Guide For Beginning Runners

Running Planet® College of Running Book Series

Rick Morris
Author of Treadmill Training for Runners

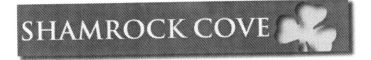

Freshman Running - A Guide for Beginning Runners

Published by:
Shamrock Cove Publishing Inc.
Post Office Box 631100
Littleton, CO 80163-1100
orders@shamrockcove.com
http://www.shamrockcove.com

Copyright © 2007 by Rick Morris
First Printing 2007

Printed in the United States of America

10 9 8 7 6 5 4 3 2 1

ISBN-13: 978-1-931088-07-7
ISBN-10 1-931088-07-1

Library of Congress Control Number: 2007906600

Notice
This book is intended as a reference only and is not intended as a replacement for professional fitness and medical advice. You should get clearance from your physician before engaging in any form of exercise. All forms of exercise pose some risks. You take full responsibility for your safety and for knowing your limits.

Mention of companies, individuals or products in this book does not imply endorsement by the publisher nor does it imply endorsement of this book by the companies or individuals mentioned.

Internet address and phone number given in this book were accurate at the time of publication

For Trish, Nika and Ripley

Forward

Running is one of the most natural and simplest acts human beings can engage in. Like the famous song by Bruce Springsteen - "We were born to run." We truly were born to run. As children we run to get around and run to play. It just came naturally. We didn't start running on the day of our birth. First we learned to crawl, then to walk and finally to run. And run we did. Just look at the kids playing outside. They run to do everything. They don't need to run, they want to. But something happened as we got older. Somewhere between childhood and adult hood many of us have forgotten how to run. We have lost the joy of running.

That is why I wrote this book. I want to bring back the joy of running. I want everyone to gain the physical and mental health benefits of running. I want you to learn to run properly so you can enjoy running for the rest of your life. That is the goal of this book.

As a running coach I have trained top level competitive runners to reach their athletic peak. Many of my athletes have gone on to reach championship levels. While I have gained great satisfaction in seeing the success of my competitive runners, I am most thrilled when I can help a new runner take the first steps in a lifetime of running. There is nothing more satisfying than seeing a new runner begin to enjoy being an athlete, improving their health and meeting goals that they never imagined they would ever be able to do. It is with that goal in mind that I bring you this training guide.

Table of Contents

"If you want to become the best runner you can be, start now. Don't spend the rest of your life wondering if you can do it."

-Pricilla Welch, masters runner

"The five S's of sports training are: stamina, speed, strength, skill and spirit; but the greatest of these is spirit."

-Ken Doherty

"Everyone is an athlete. The only difference is that some of us are in training and some are not."

-Dr. George Sheehan

Why Should You Run?

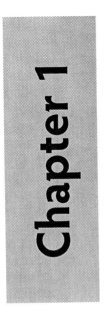

Chapter 1

A Brief History of Running

Running has been performed as a sporting activity for thousands of years, but our early ancestors ran for a very different reason - survival! Early man had to both run after their food or "prey" and run away from their predators. These distance cousins of ours could not walk down to the corner store for their groceries. They had to hunt for their food. That meant that they had to run after and chase down their dinner. At the same time, they had to protect themselves from other predators that saw them as food. They had to run away from other animals higher on the food chain. They had to run or perish!

The first "famous" runner also ran for survival. In the year 490 B.C. the Greek warrior Pheidippides ran 300 miles between the town of Marathon, Greece and Sparta in order to obtain help in defending against the invading Persians. Basic survival was his only reason for running. According to this legend, as written by the historian Herodotus in 440 B.C., Pheidippides later ran from the battlefield at

Marathon to Athens, a distance of just over 25 miles, to announce the Greek victory and proceeded to drop dead! This legend is how the modern marathon got it's name and approximate distance.

Running as a sporting event began in year 776 B.C. during the first of the ancient Olympic games in Greece. These early athletes ran for the joy of competition, fun and recreation. They also ran for the glory involved in becoming a champion. Society had advanced to the point that most people did not need to run for survival. Running had become a sport. Competition, recreation and play were the driving forces behind the development of running as a sport.

In the early to mid 1900's another reason for running became popular - health, fitness and conditioning. Arthur Lydiard was one of the first athletes to use running as a conditioning tool. Lydiard was a recreational rugby player in New Zealand in the 1940's. Looking for a way to improve his conditioning, he began a program of long slow distance running on the roads of New Zealand. At the time, the accepted method of training was to run at full speed for as long as possible. Lydiards method of long, slow distance became the backbone of today's training methods. Lydiard found that long distance running resulted in weight loss and improved conditioning. He eventually became addicted to running and entered into a career as a road racer and coach.

In the 1960's, Kenneth Cooper, an Air Force doctor, authored a book called Aerobics. This book, motivated by Cooper's health improvement obtained from running, detailed the medical reasons that an exercise program would improve health and increase life spans. This highly successful book kicked off the jogging revolution in America.

Today, people all around the world are running and participating in running events at an all-time high pace. The health, fitness and mental benefits of running are driving this new running revolution.

Physical Reasons for Running

Perhaps the most common reason for beginning a running program is to improve your physical fitness and physical health. Physical reasons include weight loss, stress reduction and cardiovascular fitness.

Weight loss and maintenance

The initial reason most athletes begin to run are physical in nature. Weight loss is the most common reason. I was a competitive runner in high school and college. After graduation, my level of training decreased to a point at which I was not maintaining my fitness level. I saw the results of this in the size of my waistline. This is what initially motivated me to begin to train consistently once again. I trained smartly and consistently. My waistline decreased to its college days size and my weight stabilized at the most healthy level for my body.

In a recent study, weight loss and weight maintenance were the most commonly reported reasons for starting an exercise program by both men and women

Running burns more calories per minute than almost any other recreational exercise. A 150-pound person, running at the moderate pace of 12 minutes per mile, burns about 10.5 calories per minute. That equals around 315 calories used during a 30 minute run. Running at a pace of 7 minutes per mile uses up calories at the blistering pace of approximately 16.8 calories per minute or over 500 calories burned in a 30 minute run. There are few methods of exercise that can match this rate of calorie burn.

Running also makes other changes in your body that increases the number of calories that you burn during the day. These changes include an increase in the number of mitochondria, which are tiny structures where the production of energy or "metabolism" of your body takes place, an increase in the number of capillaries feeding oxygenated blood to your muscles and an increase in muscle mass. Muscles are the "engines" of your body. The more muscle you have, the more calories you burn. The increased blood delivery and the increased number of mitochondria gives you a "triple whammy" that improves your body's ability to burn calories.

Running also improves your body's ability to burn fat. When your daily runs go beyond 12 to 15 minutes, more of your body fat begins to be burned as fuel. As you become more conditioned or "in shape", your body becomes more efficient at burning fat. As a result, if you run consistently, you not only burn a large amount of calories directly from the exercise, you also become a more efficient "fat burner" which makes it easier for you to lose weight or maintain your ideal body weight.

Cardiovascular fitness

Cardiovascular disease is a leading cause of premature death throughout the world. A sedentary lifestyle is one of the leading risk factors for heart attacks, stroke, hypertension (high blood pressure) and other cardiovascular problems. Any exercise that is performed continuously for 15 minutes or more and elevates your heart rate sufficiently will improve cardiovascular fitness. Running is again one the most efficient exercises at improving cardiovascular fitness.

A consistent lifelong running program will decrease your risk factors for stroke and heart problems

Depending upon your current level of fitness, you should run at an intensity that will raise your heart rate to between 50% and 95% of your maximum heart rate. You should always consult with your doctor before beginning any exercise program to determine any possible limitations to the intensity at which you should exercise. A beginning runner should not perform any highly intense workouts until a base of both aerobic fitness and strength is built.

When you are working at 50% of your maximum heart rate, you will feel like you are working at a very easy level. At 65%-70% you will feel like you are working at a comfortable, but not an easy pace. Above 70% to 75% you will start to feel like you are working hard. There is more detailed information on this in the chapter on training methods.

Heart rate training has become very popular in the last few years. However, I believe that there are many inherent problems with blindly following a heart rate monitor to adjust your training pace. Listening to your body and adjusting pace by how you are feeling is a more reliable method. Again, you will find more detailed information on this in the chapter on training methods. Whatever intensity level of exercise you need, running will easily allow you to achieve that desired level.

Runners Live Longer

When you decided to begin running you knew that running would improve your health and you probably hoped it would extend your life span. Your hope is now a fact. If you run consistently over your lifetime, a longer life span is the very probable outcome. Researchers at the University of British Columbia investigated that very topic. In that study Warbuton and associates found that sedentary individuals can prevent their risk of premature death between 20% and 50% by simply becoming more active. They also found that if you increase the amount of calories you burn through physical exercise by 1000 calories, or about 10

Recent research suggests that running just 16 miles per week may stop the advancement of cardiovascular disease and running around 22 miles per week could actually reverse the disease miles of running per week, you can reduce your risk of premature death by an additional 20%.

Strong Bones

There are 206 bones in the human body. They provide protection to your vital organs, such as your heart and brain. They provide support to the muscles so that an erect posture is possible. They provide a lever system so that the muscles can provide us with motion. They produce red blood cells and they are our "storage bins" for a number of crucial minerals.

Each of the 206 bones in your body need to be exercised to stay strong. Weight bearing activities such as running and strength training place stress on your bones which keeps them strong and healthy

Bone is composed of an organic compound called collagen, a protein that is also found in tendons and cartilage. The minerals calcium and potassium also make up bone. In 1892, Julius Wolf described how the composition of human bones are dependent upon the amount of stress that is placed upon them. The principles of Wolf's Law state that the more stress that is placed on a bone, the stronger it becomes. Conversely, reduced or lack of stress on the bone will result in a weakening of the bone. "Use it or lose it" is a common catch-phrase that describes this theory.

The bones store most of the body's supply of calcium. When dietary intake of calcium is low, the bones release calcium into the bloodstream. When dietary calcium is sufficient, the storage structures are replenished. Weakening of the bones occurs when the bones are releasing more minerals than they are taking in. A cross section of a weak bone will resemble a sponge with lots of empty cells. Bone loss can begin as early is the mid-twenties, but is usually more pronounced after 40 years of age.

One of the main risk factors for bone loss is lack of physical activity. The bones are much like the muscles. If your body senses that it does not need strong bones for activity, it does not strengthen them. If you signal your body that you need strong bones, by engaging in impact activities such as running, your body will do its best to strengthen your bones. Studies have shown that astronauts living in a zero gravity environment suffer a remarkably rapid rate of bone loss. Upon returning to normal gravity, the astronauts bones regained their previous strength. Muscle strength and bone strength seem to go hand in hand. Weight bearing exercises, including running and weight training promote the highest degree of bone strengthening.

Mental Reasons for Running

Stress Reduction

Stress has become a major health factor in today's society. The need to make more money and increased social responsibilities leaves little time for nurturing ourselves. Running has been proven to greatly reduce the levels of stress. Running reduces feelings of depression and anxiety. There are a number of documented reasons for the mental health improvements, most of which are related to the release of mood enhancing and stress reducing compounds into your bloodstream. In addition, the feeling of being in charge of your body and the feeling of being strong and conditioned is a great mood enhancer. The physical effort required for running is a great release for frustrations that build up during our daily activities.

When stresses build up, it is similar to the "fight or flight" mechanism that is instinctive in all of us. When a danger (or stressor) threatens, our heart rate increases, our blood pressure increases and hormones are released that make our muscles ready for sudden action. In our early ancestors, this would result in either a fight or flight for safety.

In today's society, our stressors are usually mental in nature and we cannot physically fight or flee. So, this stress will build up and cause mental and emotional upsets and well as potential physical problems such as cardiovascular disease. Daily physical activity, such as running, will take the place of the fight or flight mechanism and decrease the problems cause by stress.

Self Discovery and Self Improvement

I have been running competitively for over 30 years. During those years there has been a constantly increasing drive or compulsion to continue running and strive to improve myself through running. This is the one common thread among all lifelong runners. So what is the source of this inner drive? That is a difficult question that can have many answers, but it all boils down to an increase in self awareness, a desire for self improvement and plain old fun.

Your daily training run will give you the opportunity to contemplate your life, where you have been and where you are going. My training runs range from 30 minutes to over 3 hours. During that time I have designed new training strategies, planned new books, solved problems, analyzed where I have been and where I am going and just taken the opportunity to clear my mind.

As you continue your training, you will find your body fat decrease, your muscles will tighten and your energy will increase. You will feel better physically and you will mentally have more confidence in yourself. Along with a healthier, tighter and more physically fit body will become an increased awareness of where your body is in space and how it moves. You will become more fluid in your movements. You will be on your way to becoming a lifelong runner and an athlete.

You should strive to become an athlete. There is an athlete inside each one of us. Being an athlete does not necessarily mean earning your living with sports. It means working at making your body operate at its peak efficiency and pushing yourself to be your best at all times. How fast you can run or how far you can run does not matter. What matters is that you push yourself to achieve the most that you can. Running can give you a new start in life. You can rebuild your body and rid yourself of any negative thoughts and inclinations that you have had in the past. There is a lot of positive energy involved in running and racing. This energy can help make a lot of positive changes in your life.

The biological age of runners is usually significantly less than their actual age. Your biological age is a measurement of your oxygen capacity, blood pressure and ability of your body to perform physical work. A sedentary individual will usually have a biological age that is equal to or higher than their actual age. My biological age has been estimated to be 15 years less than my actual age. Biological age can be changed. If a sedentary lifestyle has given you a biological age that is higher than your actual age, a lifestyle change can reverse that.

Your actual age is your calendar age. Your biological age is a measure of the health of your cardiovascular, muscular and skeletal systems. Runners typically have younger biological ages compared to their sedentary counterparts.

In addition to a lower biological age, runners have a younger mental age. Any lifelong runner enjoys his or her chosen sport. Running is fun. A child will run for the sheer joy of running. As many of us age, the elation of running and playing gradually disappears. Why this happens is a mystery. It may be because today's society expects us to be more serious and avoid play as we age. This does not have to be so. You can still run for the joy of it. Every lifelong runner still knows the elation of running and feeling that self-generated wind blow past you. If you are going to run for the rest of your life, you must enjoy it and embrace it.

There is an appalling drop out rate in fitness and exercise programs. Over 70 percent of beginning exercisers discontinue their program and regress to their sedentary lifestyle. The main reason for this is that they simply do not enjoy it. Individuals that continue a program for life will tell you that if they do not get their workout in at some point during the day, they feel that something is missing. They will tell you that they enjoy their workout and feel energized when done. Those that drop out of an exercise program report that they do not look forward to their workouts and they feel tired when done. They feel that they are working very hard when they workout. Lifelong exercisers will tell you that they were working at a hard but enjoyable pace. So, you must enjoy what you are doing. Sometimes, when just beginning to run, you feel awkward and the act of running requires a lot of effort. This may not feel like fun to many people. Give your running program at least 6 weeks. Try to push through the times that you do not feel like running. Once your body gets in better condition, the running will become easier. You will start to feel better and will start to see results. If running is for you, you should start to enjoy it. Remember to let that child within you out to play. Have fun, there is nothing wrong with enjoying the feeling of physical activity. We all enjoyed it as a child and we can all still enjoy it now that we are older.

As your progress to higher levels of fitness, you may decide to give road racing a try. Racing gives you new opportunities to test yourself against the clock, the course and other runners. You will push yourself to even higher levels of fitness. Jogging for fitness gains and weight loss is the primary reason most people begin to run. At some point, most of us want to move on to new goals and new challenges. Racing can provide those challenges. Jogging provides great fitness benefits, but racing will give you the goal of new distances to challenge and finishing times to beat. There is no greater test of your ability to overcome challenges than that of running hard the last two miles of a 10K race or beating the overwhelming fatigue during the last 5 miles of a marathon. You will begin to feel that if you can overcome this type of challenge, you can overcome any other challenge in your life.

Other Reasons for Running

Running Can Be Done Anywhere

One of the great things about running is that it can be done almost anywhere at almost anytime, without any special equipment. Running requires no special gear, other than a good pair of running shoes. Running can be done anywhere. If you are traveling you can always find a place to run. It can be done on city sidewalks, in a park, on a beach, on a city trail, mountain trail or even on a treadmill. Running is free. There are no fees to pay or clubs to join. Running can be done alone, with a friend or with a large group. It is easy to get started. All you have to do is lace up your shoes and head out the door. If you dress appropriately, running can be done in almost any kind of weather. Rain, snow or sunshine, you will always see people out running. Many runners enjoy running in the rain.

Running Is a Good Way to Make Friends

There is a sort of camaraderie among runners. It doesn't matter whether you are a beginner or elite runner. It doesn't matter if your are old, young, big or small. All runners share a secret. It is the secret of being in control of your body, of challenging yourself everyday, of being your best, of having fun.

I run everywhere I travel and no matter where I run other runners on the trail smile and acknowledge each other. Because of this connection, running is a great way to make new friends. You may make a new friend on your daily run or you may join one of the thousands of running clubs that exist worldwide. These running clubs have organized races, social events and scheduled workouts.

Races are another way to meet other runners. If you participate in your local road races you will see the same runners over and over again. You will probably find yourself competing against the familiar faces of the runners that race at the same pace that you do. Each of the runners in these races are facing the same challenges that you are. You share a common bond with your fellow road racers. At the end of the race, be sure to congratulate your fellow runners and share your experiences. You will find they are anxious to do the same.

Improve Your Quality of Life

Perhaps the most compelling reason to run is the improvement in your quality of life. Running and other forms of exercise will almost certainly increase your life span. But even more importantly, it will improve your quality of life.

Advancements in medicine and science are continuously increasing our life spans. As we grow older, however, many of us grow weak, sick and unable to enjoy our longer life spans. Running and other forms of exercise will keep our heart, muscles, bones and mind strong are ready for the challenges of a longer life. There is no reason we must age poorly. Keep your body strong through exercise and you will enjoy every year of your life.

Are You Ready To Run?

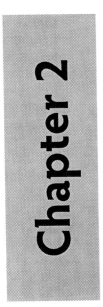

Chapter 2

Benefits Versus Risks

I hear it all the time. It's probably the comment that I get the most from non-runners. "I don't run because running is hard on your knees". Or - "You run marathons? Your knees must be pretty well shot by now. I don't know how it got started, but there is a false impression among non-runners that running is the cause of crippling knee problems and that running is hazardous for your health. Maybe the people that say those things really believe it or maybe they use if for an excuse to remain in their sedentary lifestyle. At any rate, there is nothing further from the truth. Running is one of the most efficient and fastest ways to improve your overall health, fitness and strength. If done with the proper form and mechanics, running will make your knees and legs stronger, not weaker. You will be able to run for a lifetime without any permanent joint problems if you run using proper technique.

Are there any risks at all involved in running? Of course there are. There are some risks involved in just getting out of bed. You might step on the cat and turn an ankle. You may trip over your dozing puppy and fall down the stairs. I remember one case in which then Denver Bronco's quarterback Brian Griese was injured. No - not on the field, he fell down his stairs after getting tangled up with his Golden Retriever. He missed some time and had to put up with relentless jokes in the area press, but no long term damage was done. Pets aren't the only daily hazards you could run into. You could be involved in a car accident. You might slip on snow or ice. You could burn yourself when you are cooking. I could go on and on.

My point is that everything you do involves some risk. Even if you lie in bed your entire life and never leave the house, you run the risk of developing weight and health problems from your lack of exercise. Running is no different. There are some risks that are part of any physical activity and running is no exception. You could injure a muscle. You could step on a rock or curb and turn an ankle. If you are running in the heat you could develop dehydration or heat related illnesses.

Are the risks of running higher than the risks of not running? I don't think so. I believe it is just the opposite. The risks related to lack of exercise are much higher than the risks of running. Lack of physical activity is one of the greatest risk factors involved in weight problems, cardiovascular disease and other diseases including diabetes and cancer. According to the American Heart Association, lack of physical activity has been established as a major risk factor for cardiovascular disease. They recommend that most individuals engage in at least 30 minutes of moderate intensity exercise, such as running, at least 5 days per week.

Removing risks is certainly something we should continue to try to do. But there comes a point when you cannot live a productive, healthy and satisfying life without engaging in activities that contain some small risks. Running is an example of such an activity. As with any form of physical work or exercise, there are some slight risks involved when you run. There is a chance you could become injured or ill. There are safety and health risks. What you have to consider is - do the benefits outweigh the risks involved? The benefits of running are huge and the risks are small. Here is an outline of the risks and benefits of running. You make your own decision.

Benefits

• **Improved Cardiovascular Fitness** - Your cardiovascular system is your heart, lungs and the vast network of arteries, veins and capillaries that travel throughout your body. The job of your cardiovascular system is to deliver oxygen and nutrient rich blood to the muscles and organs of your body. And conversely, the system delivers waste products to your lungs, where they are disposed of. Running or any other exercise that raises your heart rate for 15 minutes or more will improve your cardiovascular health. When you are running your muscles demand more oxygen in order to produce energy. The immediate response to those demands are met by an increased heart rate and higher stroke volume (more blood being pumped through the heart with each heartbeat). This will result in a stronger, more efficient heart muscle. Other long term improvements include decreased LDL (bad cholesterol), increased HDL (good cholesterol), lower blood pressure and slower resting heart rate.

Calories burned in 30 minutes of exercise:

Running 7 MPH - 380
Fast Swimming - 320
Tennis - 225
Basketball - 285
Golf - 184
Volleyball - 220
Walking 3.5 MPH - 160

• **Weight Loss** - Running burns more calories per minute than most any other form of exercise. Your exact rate of calorie burn will vary depending upon how fast you are running, your experience level, your running economy (a measure of how mechanically efficient you are at running) and your fitness level, but most runners average approximately 100 calories burned per mile of running. Weight loss is a function of calories in versus calories out. If you burn more calories than you are taking in, you will lose weight and body fat. So maximizing your calorie burn is critical for a weight loss or weight maintenance program. Lifelong runners will reduce their body fat content to their healthiest level and will keep it there.

• **Improved Muscle and Joint Strength** - Running is a weight bearing exercise. Any weight bearing exercise requires muscular strength. In fact, running can place anywhere between 1.5 and 4 times your own body weight on your leg muscles with each stride. That force will strengthen all of the major muscles of your hips, thighs and calf. The force required to run will also make your tendons and joints stronger. Strong tendons and joints are very important in decreasing your chance of injury.

• **Disease Prevention** - Many diseases can be prevented or the symptoms of those diseases lessened by running. Running has been show to help prevent many types of cancers, reduce the chances of developing cardiovascular diseases and help decrease the severity of the symptoms of arthritis and asthma.

• **Prevention of Osteoporosis** - Any weight bearing activity such as running and strength training has been proven to decrease the incidence of the bone loss disease, osteoporosis. Your bones are similar to your muscles in the sense that if you do not use them and place stress on them, they will weaken. "Use it or lose it" is a good axiom to follow concerning your bone heath. If you place stress on them through the use of high impact exercises, such as running and weight lifting, they will build in strength. The force generated while running strengthens your bones just as it strengthens your muscles.

• **Stress Reduction** - Running will reduce feelings of stress, depression and anxiety. The physical exertion, the release of endorphins - a mood enhancing compound and the increased confidence of having a healthy and fit body all contribute to the stress reducing benefits of running.

- **Social Benefits** - The act of training is, for the most part, a solitary activity. However, there are local races and running clubs that provide a great place to meet new friends and provide social gatherings to attend.

Risks

- **Running Injuries** - Any physical activity can result in an injury. Muscle strains, sprains, connective tissue injuries and bone injures are all possible. A beginning runner is especially susceptible to muscle strains and connective tissue injuries because the muscles and tendons are doing work that they are not used to. That is why it is important for a beginning runner to start slow and make all increases gradually. This will give your muscles and ligaments a chance to strengthen. All runners, no matter what their fitness level, will have occasional injuries. It is an unavoidable part of engaging in a healthy, physical lifestyle. When properly managed, injuries should not be a major problem

- **Physical Illness** - As well as injuries, any physical activity can result in medical conditions. Heart problems, stroke, heat and other environmentally related problems, and other medical conditions can result from any physical activity. In the vast majority of cases, running will prevent these problems. In fact, running is many times prescribed as part of a rehabilitation program for cardiac patients, but you must realize that if you have a pre-existing medical condition, any physical activity can possibly aggravate it. If you know you have a medical condition, you must consult with your doctor before beginning any exercise program.

- **Environmental Conditions** - Heat, cold, ice, snow and air pollution all present a potential hazard to runners. Running in the hot weather can be the cause of heat illnesses such as dehydration, heat exhaustion and heat stroke. Cold weather runners run the risk of hypothermia or frost bite. Working out in ice or snow can add the dangers of injury caused by slipping and falling. Running outdoors in an area of high pollution can be detrimental to your health. Air pollution can come from automobile traffic, industrial exhaust, wood burning, coal burning or even forest fires. If you suffer from asthma or any other respiratory disease, you should avoid running outside during times of high air pollution.

•   **Personal Safety** - An unfortunate risk to not only runners, but nearly everyone in today's society, is personal safety. In order to minimize this risk, you should never run alone after dark or anytime in secluded areas. Always take the steps necessary to protect yourself.

Self Health Assessment

In the past, there has been a lack of uniformity in recommendations concerning when a physical exam is necessary and what type of exercise testing should be done.

According to the American College of Sports Medicine, the minimum testing standard is the Physical Activity Readiness Questionnaire (PAR-Q). This is a questionnaire that is designed to provide individuals a way to perform a simple self assessment of their readiness to engage in an exercise program. The questionnaire asks the following seven questions:

1.   Has a doctor ever said that you have a heart condition and recommended only medically supervised activity?

2.   Do you have chest pain brought on by physical activity?

3.   Have you developed chest pain in the past month?

4.   Do you tend to lose consciousness or fall over as a result of dizziness?

5.   Do you have a bone or joint problem that could be aggravated by the proposed physical activity?

6.   Has a doctor ever recommended medication for your blood pressure or heart condition?

7.   Are you aware through your own experience, or a doctor's advice, of other physical reason against your exercising without medical supervision.

If you answered yes to one or more questions, you should consult with your doctor before beginning any exercise program. If you answered no to all questions, you are reasonably assured that you are ready for a graduated exercise program in which you make gradual increases in the level of activity. You should also get a physical exam if you any of the following apply to you:

Both traditional and non-traditional or herbal medications can have an affect on your response to exercise. Be sure to check out the possible reactions to all medications you are taking.

- Over 40 years of age.

- You are a smoker.

- You have high blood pressure.

- You have diabetes.

- You have lived a sedentary lifestyle.

- You have a family history of cardiovascular disease.

- You have high cholesterol.

Use your own common sense. If you feel that there is any possible risk at all, you should check with your doctor before you begin to run.

In addition to medical conditions, you must assess your musculoskeletal condition. If you have any prior injuries to your joints, any chronic back pain, any chronic joint pain or muscle injuries, check with your doctor before starting to run.

Effects of Medications

Some common medications can have an effect on your reaction to exercise. While the medications will not prevent your participation in exercise, you should know about the effects they cause. Talk to your doctor concerning any precautions you should take if you use medications.

•   **Beta Blockers** - This medication is prescribed for high blood pressure, migraine headaches and heart rhythm irregularities. This drug lowers your blood pressure and heart rate at rest and during exercise. You cannot use heart rate as a measure of exercise intensity if you take this medication. You should use the Borg Scale of Perceived Exertion to monitor the intensity of your workout. This scale is a rating of how hard you perceive your exercise to be. There is more information on this in the chapter on training methods.

•   **Calcium Channel Blockers** - This drug is prescribed for high blood pressure. There are several different agents available. The effect of this medication on blood pressure will vary depending upon the agent used. Check with your doctor for more information on the drug you are using.

•   **ACE Inhibitors** - This is a another medication used to lower blood pressure. ACE inhibitors block the release of a hormone that constricts the blood vessels. The effects of this drug will also vary depending upon the exact drug used. Check with your doctor if you use this medication.

•   **Diuretics** - This medication increase the excretion of water and other fluids through the kidneys. Diuretics are prescribed to lower blood pressure or in cases when a patient is accumulating too much fluid in their body. Some individuals use this drug as a weight loss aid, which is not recommended. This drug usually has no effect on heart rate.

- **Bronchodilators** - This is a medication used to treat asthma. It works by relaxing and opening the air passages in the lungs. This drug can increase both resting and exercise heart rate. This can make monitoring exercise intensity by heart rate unreliable. Use the Borg Scale of Perceived Exertion instead.

- **Decongestants** - This drug is commonly used to treat cold and flu symptoms. This medication may raise both heart rate and blood pressure. Heart rate training can be unreliable. Any exercise should be performed with caution due to the possible rise in blood pressure.

Do Runners Do Live Longer?

Imagine pulling up to the drive up window of your local drug store. You hand the pharmacist your prescription. In just a few minutes a fork lift shows up and plops a treadmill on top of your car! That's right – your doctor prescribed a treadmill to improve your health and cure your illness!

OK – Maybe I am exaggerating just a bit. You probably won't be picking up a treadmill at your neighborhood pharmacy, but more and more doctors are prescribing running and other forms of exercise to their patients. These doctors are learning what coaches, personal trainers and runners have known for years. Running is good for your physical and mental health.

As a new runner you probably assume that running will improve your health and extend your life. Your assumption is correct. If you run consistently over your lifetime, a longer life span is the very probable outcome. A study completed last year in Rotterdam confirmed that. The researchers in Rotterdam concluded that people who run about 30 minutes per day - five days per week extended their lives by 3.5 to 3.7 years. [1]

---

[1] Effects of Physical Activity on Life Expectancy With Cardiovascular Disease, Med.2005;165:2355-2360

Two Miles a Day Keeps the Grim Reaper Away

There is no question that running and other forms of physical exercise improve your health. What are the health benefits of running and how does it extend your life? Funny you should ask! Researchers at the University of British Columbia investigated that very topic in March of 2006.[2] In that study Warburton and associates found that recent research shows that sedentary individuals can reduce their risk of premature death between 20% and 50% by simply becoming more active. Even moderate amounts of running will decrease your levels of LDL (bad cholesterol), increase your HDL (good cholesterol), lower your blood pressure and improve your cardiac function. The researchers also found that if you increase the amount of calories you burn through physical exercise by 1000 calories or about 10 miles of running per week, you can reduce your risk of premature death by another 20%.

That's great news for people who are healthy and do not currently have cardiovascular disease. What about those whom are already at risk? Good news! The benefits of running also apply to individuals that already have cardiovascular disease. The researchers determined that burning around 1600 calories or 16 miles of running per week may stop the advancement of cardiovascular disease and 2200 calories or 22 miles of running per week could actually reverse the disease.

Running is a Diabetes Buster

Insulin is a hormone that your body uses to covert sugar and other foods into energy. Diabetes is a disease in which your body does not properly produce or use insulin, which can result in a dangerously high level of glucose in your blood. The most common types of diabetes are type 1 and

---

2   Health benefits of physical activity: the evidence, CMAJ March 14, 2006; 174 (6)

type 2. Type 1 diabetes is a condition in which your body fails to produce insulin. Without insulin, glucose cannot enter your cells to provide energy. Type 2 diabetes is a disease in which your body produces insulin, but you develop an insulin resistance. Your body does not properly use the insulin that is available. Most individuals diagnosed with diabetes today have type 2.

Running will help prevent the development of diabetes and also help manage existing cases. Warburton and associates found that an increase in exercise of just 500 calories per week (about 5 miles of running) will decrease the occurrence of type 2 diabetes. The study also determined physically inactive men with type 2 diabetes were 1.7 times more likely to die prematurely than physically active men with type 2 diabetes.

Running can reduce the your chances of developing colon cancer by 30% to 40%. It can decrease a women's chances of suffering from breast cancer by 20% to 30%.

Running – The Cancer Killer

There have been several studies that show that physical activity can help prevent many types of cancers, particularly colon and breast cancer. Walburton and fellow researchers reviewed over 100 studies and found that higher, more intense levels of physical activity such as running were more effective in protecting against cancer than lower level activities. They revealed that physically active men and women were 30% to 40% less likely to develop colon cancer and physically active women were at 20% to 30% less risk of developing breast cancer than their less active counterparts.

Current cancer patients can also benefit from running. One study investigated by Walburton and associates indicated that the most physically active breast cancer patients reduced their risk of cancer related death and recurrence of breast cancer by 26% to 40%.

Running Is a Bone Builder

Many critics of running will tell you that you should avoid it because it is a high impact activity. They will suggest that you should perform low-impact activities such as stationary bicycling or elliptical machines to minimize stress on your bones and joints. They are partly right but mostly wrong. They are correct that running is a high-impact activity. You are placing stress on your bones with each stride you take. They are wrong in suggesting that you should avoid all high impact exercise. Impact exercise is necessary in order to reduce the occurrence of osteoporosis. This was proven by a recent investigation that showed athletes who participate in high impact sports have higher bone density when compared to athletes who engage in low impact sports.[3]

High impact is not always a negative term. High impact exercise such as running has been proven to help build bone mass and decrease osteoporosis. A lack of impact producing exercise can increase your chances of developing osterporosis.

Your bones are similar to your muscles in the fact that a lack of stress will result in weakness. If you do not exercise your muscles they will atrophy or get smaller and weaker. The same principle applies to your bones. If your bones are not consistently stressed, they will become weak and brittle. If you consistently stress them through high impact activities such as running or strength training, they will respond by growing stronger. Warburton and associates found that running 15 to 20 miles per week is associated with maintaining or building bone density. Another study conducted in the year 2000 showed that intense physical activity led to a reduced incidence of hip fractures in the men studied.[4]

---

3   The effects of changes in musculoskeletal fitness on health. Can J Appl Physiiol 2001;26:161-216

4   Physical activity and osteoporotic hip fracture risk in men. Arch Intern Med 2000;160:705-8

Exercise also helps decrease the severity of existing osteoporosis. In a 6 month study, 98 older women with osteoporosis participated in high impact exercise training. The exercise improved their bone densities by .5% to 1.4%.[5]

How Far Should You Go?

As you can see there is no doubt that running will improve your health, increase your level of fitness and probably extend your life, but how far should you run? The answer to that question depends upon your current situation. Any amount of exercise will help. While most fitness professionals recommend a minimum weekly energy expenditure of 1000 calories (10 miles of running), burning as little as 500 calories (5 miles of running or walking) per week has been shown to be beneficial to your health. This is especially true for individuals who have been sedentary, have very low fitness levels, the frail or elderly. But there is also evidence that a much higher volume and intensity of exercise is more beneficial.

Berkeley researcher Paul Williams and assistant Davina Moussa conducted a study of 1,833 women as part of the National Runners Health Study. The study investigated the benefits of prolonged running. Williams and Moussa determined that running more miles resulted in greater health benefits, up to 40 miles per week. Running over 40 miles per week will continue to improve your level of fitness, but the researchers found that there were few health or life extension benefits obtained from running more than 40 miles per week.

Is There a Dark Side?

One of my favorite movies when I was young was the original Star Wars. A part of that movie that has stayed with me over the years is the eerie scene involving the heavy and raspy breathing of Darth Vader, who represented the dark side.

5   J Clin densitom 2004;7:390-8

Running provides many physical and mental health benefits, but is there a dark side to running? Some believe that there is. Occasionally a tragedy occurs in the sport of running. Runners that appear to be fit and healthy collapse and die during their race or training run. During the 2006 Los Angeles Marathon two men died after suffering a heart attack. One runner suffered a heart attack 3 miles into the race while the other collapsed at mile 21. A third runner had a heart attack at the start of the race but survived.

A recent study showed the the risk of sudden death among marathon runners is .002% which is much lower that a group of non-runners.

Sudden death is not a common occurrence in running, even during a race as grueling and strenuous as the marathon. It is even rarer to see multiple deaths, such as the unfortunate events during the 2006 Los Angeles Marathon, but sudden deaths do occur. Studies vary in data concerning the number of sudden deaths among runners. One report said that about 7 of every 100,000 runners will die suddenly. Another recent study determined that sudden death associated with moderate to vigorous exercise was very low at 1 per 36.5 million hours of exercise.[6] In 2005, researchers conducted a study of 215,413 runners that competed in the Marine Corp and Twin Cities Marathons over a 30 year period.[7] The researchers found that only 4 sudden deaths occurred due to unsuspected heart disease. That is a very low .002% which is much lower than risks of sudden death among non-runners. Regardless of which numbers you choose to believe, the incidence of sudden death among runners is rare.

Sudden death during exercise is a relatively rare occurrence, but unfortunately it does happen. If running and ex-

---

6   Physical exertion, exercise and sudden cardiac death in women. JAMA 2006;295:1399-1403

7   J.Am.Coll,Cardiol.2005;46;1371-1374

ercise improves your health and extends your life, why do these tragedies happen? Does running increase the chances of sudden death? As with most complex questions, the answer is partly yes and partly no.

This question became a full blown controversy in the early 1980's with the death of running author Jim Fixx. Fixx became famous as the writer of the international best selling book "The Complete Book of Running". This was one of the first books to introduce the joys and benefits of running to the general population and was credited for helping fuel the running boom of the 1980's. Fixx died of a heart attack while running and immediately the blame for his sudden death fell upon running and vigorous exercise.

The most common cause of death in today's society is coronary artery disease. Almost every investigation agrees; nearly all runners that die suddenly during exercise already had advanced cardiovascular disease. None of these diseases are caused by running. It has been proven time and time again that running and other forms of exercise help prevent heart disease. A runner with heart disease is more like to suffer from a fatal heart attack when exercising than when at rest. This makes sense because the strain on the heart is obviously greater during strenuous exercise. However, because of the health benefits of exercise, if those same runners were to avoid exercise, their risk of sudden death at all times would rise, not fall.

The death of Jim Fixx is a perfect example of this. Fixx already had heart disease at the time of his death. He was a former smoker and had a family history of heart disease. His father had died of a heart attack at age 43. Fixx also had elevated blood cholesterol. Three of his coronary arteries were blocked, one at 95%, one at 85% and one at 50%. He died at age 53, outliving his father by 10 years. Running did not kill Jim Fixx. On the contrary, it almost certainly allowed him to live a longer, happier and more productive life.

Run On

There is not a doubt in the world that habitual, consistent runners live longer, healthier and happier lives. Running helps prevent, manage and reduce cardiovascular disease, diabetes, arthritis, osteoporosis, cancer and other diseases. It keeps your weight at a healthy level, lowers your blood pressure, reduces bad cholesterol, increases good cholesterol, builds your strength and improves your cardiac function. Running also reduces your stress level, anxiety and depression.

Runners that already have heart disease are slightly more at risk of sudden death during exercise than when they are at rest, but without exercise their risk of sudden death is greater at all times. If you currently have, or have a family history of, cardiovascular disease, high blood pressure, high cholesterol, if you are a smoker or if you are over 50 you should be screened by your doctor before you begin or continue running.

Running is good for you and data shows that it will add years to your life. So run on. Runners do live longer.

Your Body In Action

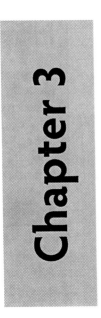

Your body is a remarkable biological machine. It will do its best to do what you ask it to do and will strengthen itself in order to do so. This is, in essence, what a fitness or sports training program really is. It is the process of asking your body to do more than it is accustomed to and your body responds by getting stronger. When you begin running for the first time your body says - "What the heck is this person doing? We have never been asked to this before!" In response your muscles, joints and connective tissues become stronger, fitter and more capable of providing you with a runner's body.

You don't need to be a professional coach or an exercise physiologist in order to train yourself. However, it will help to have a basic understanding of how your body moves, produces the energy required for movement and how it responds to training. The amount material you would need to read in order to understand everything about your body's physiology would fill a small truck, but here are the fundamentals that will give you a basic understanding of your body in action.

How Muscles Work

Muscles are made up of thousands of small individual muscle fibers. Imagine a large rope. The rope is made up of many small fibers. Each fiber individually is very weak and could be easily broken. But, there is strength in numbers. When the many individual rope fibers are joined together, they make up a very strong length of rope. Your muscles are very similar to this. Each individual muscle fiber is relatively weak. But, just as the rope, when many fibers are joined together you have a very strong muscle. The larger, more powerful muscles in your body have more individual fibers. For example, the muscles in your pinkie finger are small compared to your thigh muscles. The large muscles of your thigh are made up of many muscle fibers and you are able to use them to run, jump, ski and many other activities that require a large amount of strength. On the other hand, your pinkie has relatively few muscle fibers. Your pinkie is strong enough to allow you to type, eat or turn the pages of a book, but just imagine if you tried to support all of your weight on that one little finger. It would instantly collapse.

Your muscles are made up of many small, individual muscle fibers, much like the strands of a rope. Larger muscles have more strands or fibers and are much stronger.

Each muscle fiber is essentially composed of a series of overlapping proteins. When a signal is sent to your muscle to contract or shorten, these proteins pull against each other, which result in a contraction of the muscle. That shortening or contraction of the muscle results in movement. This is a very simplified description of a highly complicated process, but it will work for our purposes here.

Every movement you make and every muscle you move is accomplished by a signal sent from your brain to the muscle that is moving. The signal is sent from your brain to a motor unit in the muscle. A motor unit is composed of a nerve ending and the number of muscle fibers that the nerve controls. Motor units comes in many sizes. It may control only a few muscle fibers or it may control hundreds. The force of the muscle contraction depends upon how many motor units are called into action. For instance the act of picking up a piece of cotton with your finger will use only a few motor units. Picking up a heavy weight or running at full speed uses many motor units. This process is important in understanding how your body strengthens and improves with physical training.

All movements start in your brain, where a signal is sent to the motor units in your muscles instructing them to activate your muscle

Muscle Fiber Types

You have noticed that some athletes can run very fast but not vary far, while others can run very far but are not good at sprinting. One of the reasons for this is the athletes percentage of two types of muscle fibers.

There are two basic types of muscle fibers. They are called **slow twitch** muscle fibers and **fast twitch** muscle fibers. They acquired their names simply because the slow twitch fibers contract more slowly and the fast twitch fibers contract faster.

We all have both types of fibers in our body. The percentage of each type will differ from person to person. The percentage of each is genetically determined. It is something we are born with and, for the most part, cannot be changed. The slow twitch fibers contract more slowly, but are more fatigue resistance. The fast twitch fibers contract faster and more forcefully, but are quick to fatigue. A world class marathon runner will likely have 75 to 98 percent slow twitch muscle fibers. In contrast, a top level sprinter may have 75 to 80 percent fast twitch muscle fibers.

I mentioned earlier that, for the most part, you cannot change your muscle fiber type. Research has shown that is the case. However, you can make your fast twitch fibers a little bit more resistant to fatigue with proper training. That is one of the reasons that you are able to run further without fatigue as you progress through your training program.

How Energy Is Produced

Now you know the basics of how muscles produce movement. In order to produce that movement the muscles need energy and lots of it. Your body completes many highly complex chemical reactions to produce all of that energy. So you don't have to wade through a 500 page biology textbook I will break the process down into a simple concepts. Here are the basics of energy production.

ATP

ATP is an abbreviation for adenosine triphosphate. Simply put, ATP is a substance that is your body's energy source, much as gasoline is the energy source for your gas powered automobile. Without ATP, your muscles will not work. How quickly and efficiently your body can produce ATP determines how quickly your muscles reach fatigue.

There are three ways that your body produces ATP. They are commonly called the aerobic system, the anaerobic system and the creatine phosphate system. Aerobic means "with oxygen". The aerobic system depends upon a sufficient delivery of oxygen to your muscles cells. Anaerobic means "without oxygen. Both the anaerobic and the creatine phosphate system will work without the presence of oxygen.

Creatine Phosphate Energy Production

The simplest way to produce ATP is with the creatine phosphate system. This system uses a substance to produce energy very quickly. This substance is called phosphocreatine. The energy from phosphocreatine is not directly used to energize the muscles. The energy from this molecule is used to produce ATP, which does directly supply energy to make your muscles work. This process works very quickly and without oxygen. The problem with this system is the limited supply of the phosphocreatine.

There is only enough of this substance to energize your muscles for 5 to 20 seconds of work. This system is used for the first few seconds of a very intense activity such as sprinting and heavy weight lifting. It is not a major contributor to energy production for long distance runners. Competitive distance runners will sometimes draw on this energy producing system during the final all out sprint to the finish line.

The average runner can only store about 50 grams of ATP in their muscle cells. A sedentary person needs a whopping 190,000 grams just to meed their daily needs. If you are an active runner you need much more.

Anaerobic Energy Production

The word anaerobic means "without oxygen". When you are exercising at an intense level your muscles require large amounts of energy and they need it very quickly. At high running speeds, your cells are not able to extract enough oxygen from your blood to produce energy aerobically. In that case, the anaerobic system begins to dominate the energy production in your body.

The anaerobic system uses glucose to produce ATP. Glucose is the storage form of sugars in your body and bloodstream. The glucose comes from digestion of carbohydrates you have eaten and from stores of glycogen (converted glucose) in your muscles and liver. The process of making ATP from glucose is a very complex series of chemical reactions. I will spare you the gory details. One important thing to remember is that the conversion of glycogen into ATP results in a by-product called pyruvic acid. This compound is then converted into another compound called lactic acid.

Most of your energy is produced either aerobically or anaerobically, but never exclusively. When you are running slowly most energy is produced aerobically. As you speed up, more energy is produced using the anaerobic system, but both systems are always being utilized.

Your body is able to use the lactic acid to produce more energy. At moderate paces, all of the lactic acid is cleared and converted into energy. The faster you run, the more quickly lactic acid is produced. Eventually, you begin to produce lactic acid faster than your body can process it and a backlog of lactic acid begins to build up. The build up of lactic acid eventually causes your blood be become more acidic due to an accumulation of hydrogen ions. The acidity levels in your blood eventually reach a point at which further conversion of glucose to ATP is inhibited and the muscles ability to work is decreased. This is believed to be one of the major limiting factors with the anaerobic system.

Another limiting factor with both the anaerobic system and the creatine phosphate system is the relatively small amount of ATP that is produced. When the anaerobic system is used, the muscles reach fatigue in approximately 1 to 5 minutes. You will know when you are working anaerobically because you will be hyperventilating or breathing at a very rapid and heavy pace. This is caused by your body attempting to force more oxygen into your system in order to produce energy aerobically. However, your rate of breathing does not limit energy production. It is your cells ability to extract oxygen from your blood that is the limiting factor, so all that heavy breathing is, for the most part, an exercise in futility.

Aerobic Energy Production

In opposition to anaerobic, aerobic means "with oxygen" This system for producing ATP dominates when a sufficient supply of oxygen is available to the muscle cells. This system uses both glucose (carbohydrates) and fats to produce ATP. The percentage of glucose and fat used depends upon the intensity of the exercise. At rest and at lower intensity, more fat is burned than glucose. As the intensity increase, more and more glucose is used.

This continues up to the level at which your body is unable to find enough oxygen to support the aerobic system. This level is called the anaerobic threshold or lactate threshold. A more accurate description may be lactate turn point. Above this level, your body will depend more on the anaerobic system or the creatine phosphate system. This is sometimes known as the lactate threshold because it is the point at which lactic acid (which is converted into a compound called lactate) begins to accumulate in your blood.

Your muscles need an adequate supply of oxygen in order to produce energy aerobically. The aerobic energy production system completely breaks down both carbohydrates and fats to produce ATP

It is important to realize that there is not a single point at which your body switches from strictly aerobic energy production to just anaerobic energy production. You are always using both systems. Even when you are resting, there is some anaerobic energy production going on. As you increase the intensity of your running you begin to rely more and more on the anaerobic system. Your lactate threshold is the point at which your blood become so acidic that you aerobic system can no longer dominate and your anaerobic system becomes the predominate system. In other words, you aerobic system is still working full time, but has become "maxed out" and your anaerobic system must pick up the slack and take over.

The aerobic production of ATP results in the same by-product as the anaerobic system - pyruvic acid. The difference in the aerobic system is that instead of then being converted in lactic acid, which limits performance, the pyruvic acid goes through another energy producing system called the Krebs Cycle. This produces an additional amount of ATP. This aerobic system produces much more ATP than the other two systems, but requires large amounts of oxygen in order to work.

Aerobic energy production takes place inside tiny structures called mitochondria. This substance is located in most cells, but especially in muscle cells. Anaerobic and creatine phosphate energy production takes place inside the cells, but outside the mitochondria. This rather obscure detail will be important to remember when we discuss the reasons your body improves its performance in response to proper training.

Why You Become Fatigued

Fatigue is an unavoidable part of running. You will only avoid feelings of fatigue on your easy run days. Even on those easy run days, you may reach low levels of fatigue.

The feelings of fatigue will vary greatly. What fatigue feels like after a 15 second sprint is very different than what you feel like in the last miles of a marathon. The causes of fatigue are just as diverse. The most common causes of fatigue are related to one of the following:

•　　Energy production systems (aerobic, anaerobic, creatine phosphate)

•　　Rise in the acidity of your blood (lactic acid)

•　　Neuromuscular fatigue (transmission of signals to your muscles)

These common causes are all physical causes of fatigue. There are also a number of causes of day to day fatigue, such as stress, lack of proper sleep, poor nutrition and emotional upset. Since a complete discussion of all possible causes of fatigue would fill volumes, we will concentrate on the common physical causes that are directly related to running.

Energy System Fatigue

Phosphocreatine Depletion

Remember phosphocreatine, the source of short term, highly intense energy? The supply of this substance, in your body, is very limited. This system produces ATP for short, intense bursts of energy. The supply of creatine phosphate will be depleted within 5 to 20 seconds. When the creatine phosphate supply is gone, your production of ATP is also gone, until its production is picked up by another system. This is the cause of fatigue when performing an all out sprint. You simply will not be able to continue after your supply of phosphocreatine is gone.

When performing sprinting events of longer than 20 seconds, such as 200 meter or 400 meter sprints, you must learn to pace your self in the early stages of the race. If you start out too fast you will deplete both your phosphocreatine supply and your ATP supplies and you will be unable to hold your pace in the final portions of the race.

Glycogen Depletion

When you eat foods containing carbohydrates, your digestive system converts the various sugars in the carbohydrates into glucose. This conversion is necessary to make the carbohydrates usable by your body. When the glucose is released into your bloodstream a hormone called insulin is also released. Insulin tells your body's tissues to store some of the newly released glucose. This is stored in your muscle and liver as glycogen. Glycogen is glucose molecules that are linked together and is the storage form of glucose.

In very brief bursts of high speed, the creatine phosphate system is used. In events lasting longer than approximately 20 seconds, the anaerobic system, which uses glucose to produce ATP, is used. This system will last from around 1 minute to 5 minutes depending upon the intensity of the exercise. This system will be used primarily for races from 400 meters to 1600 meters. Glycogen stores in the muscles are limited and are depleted quickly. Just as with shorter sprints, you must learn to properly pace yourself in order to prevent glycogen depletion before the end of your race.

Glycogen depletion is also a factor in the aerobic energy production system. The aerobic system is used when you are running at a pace at which your body can extract sufficient oxygen from your blood to support the system. This system dominates during longer races such as 2 miles up to marathons. The aerobic system uses glycogen at much lower rate for two reasons. The intensity of the exercise is lower, so less is used. The aerobic system also uses fat and the conversion of pyruvic acid for ATP production, so this lessens the demand for glycogen.

The marathon term "hitting the wall" refers to the extreme fatigue caused by a combination of glycogen depletion and neuromuscular fatigue.

Glycogen depletion is one of the main causes of fatigue for marathon runners. During marathon pace runs, your stores of glycogen will be depleted at around 18 to 21 miles (29 to 35 km). This point is referred to, by marathoners, as "hitting the wall". Much of this sensation is caused by a nearly complete depletion of glycogen.

Fatigue From Blood Acidity

Remember earlier I said that a by-product of anaerobic energy production is lactic acid? There is a very common misconception that this accumulation of lactic acid is the cause of all muscle fatigue. Lactic acid accumulation is a factor in fatigue only during short to moderate length events and highly intensity events, such as short sprints, 5K and 10K races. During longer races lactic acid actually becomes an additional source of ATP production. Even in the shorter events, the presence of lactic acid is not the direct cause of fatigue. Without getting too technical (you can thank me later), the lactic acid goes through a conversion that results in the accumulation of hydrogen ions. The hydrogen ions cause a condition called acidosis. This condition causes your body to release buffers that reduce the effect of the hydrogen ions. The end result is that the buffers cause a decrease in the muscle pH, which causes a decrease in the ability of your muscles to do work.

Lactic acid has gotten a bad rap over the years. It has received the blame for a whole slew of problems from muscle soreness and stiff muscles to the primary cause of fatigue. Now we know that not only is lactic acid not the cause of those problems, but is in fact, a valuable source of energy.

Some exercise physiologists believe that this process is a caused by your body trying to protect itself. If the acids in your muscle were allowed to continue to rise, serious muscle damage could be the result. The buffers that decrease your muscles ability to work could be a self protective mechanism that keeps you from damaging your body by continuing to run at an intense pace when your muscles are already too acidic.

Potassium Buildup Fatigue

Many researchers now believe that potassium build up rather than lactic acid accumulation is a primary cause of running fatigue. There is even some data that shows lactic acid can actually reduce the effects of potassium build up and improve running endurance.

A recent and interesting finding is that a buildup in potassium can also be a major contributor to running fatigue. Your muscles depend upon an exchange between potassium and sodium to fire a muscle contraction. During high intensity distance running potassium is released faster than it can be used. This can cause an interruption or weakening of the ability of your muscles to contract - or in simpler terms, it causes fatigue. This potassium build up takes place at roughly the same pace and at the same time as the hydrogen ion build up, so it is difficult to determine whether the hydrogen ion build up or the potassium is causing the fatigue. The most recent research[1] seems to point to potassium build up, but both probably play a role.

Neuromuscular Fatigue

Another possible source of fatigue involves a disruption of the signals sent from your brain to your exercising muscles. There is some new evidence that suggests that a number of chemical reactions can take place that reduces the ability of the signal receptors in the motor units to receive the signal and also reduces the muscles ability to contract. More research needs to be done in this area to prove or disprove these theories. This type of fatigue may also be a self protective mechanism.

---

1   Potassium, Na+,K+ pumps and muscle fatigue. J Physiol 2007 Aug 2

How Your Body Improves With Training

Your body reacts to the stress or lack of stress that is placed upon it. If you are engaging in an exercise program that places progressively higher levels of stress on your muscles and cardiovascular system, those systems grow stronger. If you stop exercising for a long period of time your body will react to that in a similar way. Your muscles no longer need to be strong so they begin to weaken and become less fit. A proper training program will make improvements in both your muscular strength and cardiovascular conditioning or metabolic function. All improvements are necessary in order to maximize your running performance. Strength is not only improved in your muscles, but also in your connective tissues (tendons, cartilage), joints and bones. Your neuromuscular conditioning is also improved. Your neuromuscular system involves the ability of your brain to communicate quickly and efficiently with your muscles. It is like installing new high speed phone lines from your brain to your muscles. If you have switched from dial up internet access to high speed access you have experienced a similar change. The lines from your brain to your muscles make a similar change from slow and sluggish to lightning fast speed.

The old axiom "use it or lose it" is an accurate way to describe your body's reaction to training. Training is very simple. If you place stress on your muscle, joints and bones, they grow stronger in response. If you take away the stress, they know the additional strength is no longer needed and they grow weaker.

Strength Improvements

Muscle Fibers

A strength training program or a weight bearing cardio-vascular exercise, such as running, will cause an increase in the size of the muscle itself. This is called hypertrophy. The increase in size is caused mostly by an increase in the size of the muscle fibers and an increase in muscle protein, not an increase in the number of fibers. There is some controversy concerning whether or not it is possible to increase the number of muscle fibers. Some research has shown that lifting very heavy weights can increase the number of fibers, but this research is inconclusive at this point.

Connective Tissue

Proper training will also increase the strength of your connective tissue. There are three types of connective tissue in your body. **Cartilage** is a type of padding that provides cushioning and lubrication between two moving joints. The most important cartilage for runners is the cartilage in the knee joint. **Ligaments** are tissues that connect bones together at a joint. **Tendons** are tissues that connect the muscles to the bones.

Your body will try to do what ever you ask it to do. When your connective tissue is put under more stress than it is accustomed to, it will strengthen itself in response. This increase in connective tissue strength will help you prevent injures and also plays a large role in overall strength gains.

Neural Activity

The initial gains in strength are not due to muscle size increase or connective tissue strength gains. It is due to an increase in the number of motor units that are operating. Remember from earlier, that the motor units receive the signals from your brain to contract the muscles. The more motor units that are operating, the more muscles contract and the stronger you become. An untrained person has fewer motor units operating than a trained person. These dormant motor units respond very quickly and become active with proper training.

The first noticable fitness gains are usually due to improvements in your neural activity or the ability of your brain to communicate with your muscles.

Metabolic Function

Your body's level of cardiovascular conditioning is really a measure of your metabolic function. Your metabolism is basically the utilization of energy. Both anaerobic and aerobic training will improve your metabolic function.

Aerobic Training

Remember that the aerobic system is used when there is a sufficient supply of oxygen to the cells. Aerobic training uses this system. Your daily training runs, with the exception of high intensity speed work and lactate threshold workouts, are aerobic workouts. There are five major adaptations that your body makes in response to aerobic exercise. These are muscle adaptations, capillary density, amount of myoglobin in your blood, mitochondria density and the production of aerobic enzymes.

•   **Muscle adaptations** to strength training were discussed earlier. Aerobic training also makes improvements in muscles. Recall that we all have a combination of slow twitch and fast twitch muscles. I mentioned that you cannot change your muscle types, but you can make your fast twitch fiber more fatigue resistant. There are actually two types of fast twitch fibers. They are called fast twitch a (FTa) and fast twitch b (FTb). FTb fibers are quicker to fatigue than FTa fibers. Long term aerobic training has been shown to change the characteristics of the FTb fibers so that they are a bit more resistant to fatigue, much as the FTa fibers.

•   **Capillary density** increases with aerobic training. Capillaries are the very small blood vessels that transfer oxygen to the muscle cells. More capillaries means more blood flow and oxygen delivery to the muscle cells. Endurance training has been shown to increase the number of capillaries by as much as 15%.

•   **Myoglobin** is a compound in your blood that attaches to oxygen and transfers the oxygen into the mitochondria. Recall that the mitochondria is where the aerobic energy production takes place. Endurance training greatly increases the amount of myoglobin in your blood. Myoglobin has been shown to increase by as much as 80% in response to training. More myoglobin in your blood will allow more oxygen to reach your muscles. That means you will be fitter and able to run both further and faster.

•   **Mitochondria** density also increases in response to aerobic training. Since aerobic energy production takes place in the mitochondria, it follows that more mitochondria will provide more potential to produce energy. Training will increase both the number of mitochondria in the cells and the size of the mitochondria. This is one of the most critical factors in your fitness and endurance levels.

•   **Aerobic enzymes** are necessary in order to facilitate the breakdown of fuels and the production of ATP.

Enzyme activity increases by 25% with moderate amounts of exercise and up to 250% with daily vigorous exercise. Those numbers illustrate the importance of consistent daily exercise.

Anaerobic Training

• **Anaerobic enzymes** are increased by anaerobic training. Just as aerobic training increases aerobic enzyme activity, anaerobic training increases anaerobic enzyme activity. These enzymes are required in order to produce ATP using the anaerobic or creatine phosphate systems. You are training anaerobically when your are running at high intensity paces that can only be continued for 1 to 5 minutes.

• **Lactate threshold** or anaerobic threshold is the level at which your body can no longer supply enough oxygen to your muscle cells in order to maintain use of the aerobic energy system. Remember that at this level lactic acid begins to accumulate in your blood. By training at this anaerobic threshold level, you will train your body to become better at buffering and clearing this lactic acid from your blood, which will result in better performance and overall fitness.

• **Running economy** is a measure of the efficiency of your running form and style. Fast paced running will improve your balance, coordination and strength when running. Your running will become more economical, allowing you to run with less effort, using less energy. If you are a more efficient runner you will also be able to avoid many common running injuries.

What To Wear

Choice of clothing can have a positive or negative influence on how much you enjoy your run and can even affect your health and safety. There is a large selection of running clothing available. Most of the items made especially for runners will do the trick, but what you should wear will depend upon where you are running and what the weather is like.

We all want to look our best at all times. Don't choose your running outfit with only appearance in mind. Dress functionally for comfort and safety, not for fashion.

As a general rule, if the weather is moderate, you should wear light, loose fitting clothes when you run. You don't want to wear anything that will interfere with your running stride. A good choice would be lightweight shorts and a light porous top. Cotton will absorb sweat and allow it to evaporate slowly but can also absorb and hold a lot of moisture next to your body. There are a number of special synthetic fabrics that are very good at wicking sweat away from your body.

Dressing for Hot Weather Running

When running in hot weather it is important to keep your body as cool as possible. The first rule is not to overdress. You body cools itself through the evaporation of sweat. If you overdress some of the heat will be trapped and you could overheat in even mild temperatures.

You should wear clothes that are light and loose. Some runners like to run shirtless or with just a sports bra. While that will keep you cool, it is sometimes a better idea to wear some covering to prevent sunburn. Long-term exposure to the UV rays from the sun has been shown to cause premature skin aging and skin cancer. Be sure to apply sweat proof sunscreen to all of your exposed skin surfaces when running in the hot sun.

Shirts and Shorts

Clothing that is made from cotton will absorb a lot of sweat from your body. The problem with cotton is that the moisture continues to collect and you end up wearing a soaking wet shirt. There are a number of special synthetic fabrics that are designed to wick moisture away from the skin and allow it to evaporate slowly. This type of fabric will keep you cool and will also avoid that soaking wet feeling and the skin chafing that sometimes accompanies it.

Socks

A lot of running socks are 100% cotton socks and suffer from the same problem as shirts and shorts. The cotton will absorb a lot of moisture. That trapped moisture will make your feet wet, uncomfortable and can result in the formation of blisters. Socks are available that are made from the same synthetic fibers as shirts and shorts. That type of sock will help keep your feet dry and comfortable.

Running socks are available both with or without padding. If you do not have problems with foot pain or blisters, the lightweight socks without padding are the best bet. If blisters are a problem or if your feet become uncomfortable during your run, you might give the padded socks a try.

Many runners prefer to run with no socks because their feet stay cooler. For most runners, the socks provide an extra bit of cushioning and comfort. Try it both ways and go with the method that feels best to you, but be cautious with going sockless. It makes your feet more vulnerable to blisters.

Outer Wear

Many new runners make the mistake of wearing a warm up suit or sweat suit while running. They believe that the additional sweat produced will burn off more fat. This is not correct. The excessive sweat will only dehydrate you which can lead to the dangerous condition of heat exhaustion or even heat stroke, which can be fatal. Only the burning of calories through exercise will reduce body fat. It is very important to wear clothing that will keep you cool, when running in hot weather. Any type of clothing that traps heat should be avoided.

Dressing for Cold Weather Running

When running in cold weather, remember one word - layers. Always dress in layers. Layers will provide you with a lot of flexibility. The layers will keep you warm by trapping heat against your body. During your run you will begin to generate a lot of heat. If you become overheated you can remove layers.

I would recommend wearing either two or three layers depending upon how cold it is. The purpose of the first layer is to wick the moisture away from your skin. A long sleeve cotton shirt will wick the moisture away, but will also hold onto that moisture. Eventually it will become saturated and could cause you to become chilled. A better choice for the first layer would be an acrylic fabric, polypropylene or any of the new high tech fabric that are designed to keep the moisture away from your skin. The second layer is the one that should trap the heat in. It should be made of an insulating material such as fleece or heavy cotton. It should also be able to absorb a bit of moisture, since it will be covering your first, wicking layer.

Each layer of clothing has a specific purpose.

Layer 1 - The inner layer wicks moisture away from your skin.

Layer 2 - The middle layer insulates your body and keeps you warm.

Layer 3 - The outer layer breaks the wind and keeps you dry.

During moderately cold and dry weather, you may only need two layers. If it is extremely cold, raining, snowing or windy, you should wear a third layer. This layer is needed to break the wind and keep you dry. It also adds an additional insulating factor in very cold weather. This outer layer should be made of a waterproof material such as Gortex or nylon.

One rule of thumb to follow is that you should be a little bit cold when you start. As you run and generate body heat you will warm up. If you are comfortable when you start, you will probably become overheated later on. If you do become overheated, you can either unzip your outer layer or remove a layer completely.

Cool to Moderate Weather - 40 to 65 degrees Fahrenheit

This is the most difficult weather to dress for. A single layer of clothing is the best bet. Wear either a long sleeve or short sleeve shirt depending upon the exact temperature and your personal comfort level. Shorts are usually warm enough for these conditions. If you prefer a bit more warmth, you could wear lightweight tights. Running gloves and a headband or hat will provide some added warmth, especially if it is windy. If it is raining, wear a water resistant outer nylon shell. You will probably feel a bit cold when you first start running, but you will soon generate enough body heat to keep you warm.

Cold Weather - 15 to 39 degrees Fahrenheit

You will want to wear at least two layers of clothing in cold weather. Start with a long sleeve shirt and heavy weight running tights. Add a water resistant running jacket for the outside layer. You will definitely want running gloves and a headband or hat. You lose a lot of body heat through your head in cold weather.

Very Cold Weather - Below 15 degrees Fahrenheit

In this severe weather, you will want three layers. Start with a long sleeve shirt and tights made of a wicking fabric. Add an insulating long sleeve shirt and heavy weight running pants as the second layer. Use a water resistant running jacket as the third layer. If the weather is wet, you could also add some water resistant pants. Make sure you wear running gloves, insulating hat and perhaps a heavy weight scarf.

Running In The Rain

Singing in the Rain is one of the all time classic movies. And of course the most famous scene from that movie is of Gene Kelly dancing and singing in the rain. He was having a great time. Running in the rain can be the same. If the weather is warm running in the rain can be very fun and refreshing. I remember one year I was in Orlando, Florida for the Disney World Marathon. A couple of days before the race I was doing a short run and the sky opened up. I have never seen it rain so hard. But, it was a hot day and the rain felt like a warm, heavy shower. I was soaked, but it was one of the most enjoyable runs I ever had. My point is that there is nothing wrong with running in the rain during warm weather. If you do run in the rain, wear a light weight wicking fabric. Cotton will hold onto every rain drop and will become very heavy and clinging. The wicking fabrics will stay light on your skin. Also try to wear a spare pair of running shoes. Your shoes will become very saturated and may not dry out in time for your next run.

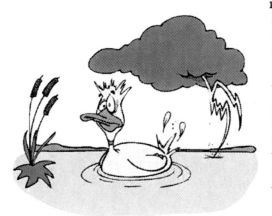

If you are caught out in the open during a lightning storm you could be a "sitting duck". Don't take a chance. If there is lightning in the area, run inside on your treadmill or wait for the storm to pass.

Running in a cold rain is another story. You can become chilled very quickly and even put yourself at risk of developing hypothermia if you are not properly dressed. Always wear an outside waterproof layer to keep the cold rain from reaching your inside layer and your skin. If it is cold enough that you are wearing running tights, you should also put on a pair of water proof pants.

Many summer rain storms will also include lightning. This is something that you do not want to mess with. If there is any lightning in the area, do not run outside. It is time to hit the treadmill during this kind of weather. Even if the lightning seems to be in the distance, do not go out for a run. The lighting can move in quickly or a rogue bolt can come out of nowhere. I learned my lesson the hard way. One day I was heading out for my daily run on a small ridge near my house. There was a storm moving in, but it appeared to be far to the west. I saw some lightning, but seemed to be very distant. I got to the top of the ridge, about 2 miles from my house, when a lightning bolt came out of nowhere. It missed me, but needless to say I set a two mile record on the way back to my house. Now I either stay on the treadmill or wait until the storm passes.

Dressing for Races

Dressing for a race presents it own special challenges. Many races will start early in the morning when the temperature may be low. In short races, such as 5K's or 10K's, wear clothing that is appropriate for the expected weather. Watch the local weather forecast the night before the race. If the weather is going to be cool at start time, take along a warm-up suit. Keep the suit on until just before race time. If you have anyone with you that will be watching the race, give the suit to them for safekeeping. If you are alone, you will want to

Plan to slightly under dress for races and training runs. You should feel slightly cold before you start. If you are warm before you start you will probably be over heated during your race or run

allow enough time to take the suit back to your car before the race starts. Do not overdress. You will be running at a hard pace during the race and you will generate a lot of body heat. Plan on being a bit cold at the start.

If you are running a longer race, such as a marathon, you will want to dress in layers. In the bigger marathons, there will be a tent or bus at which you can drop your warm up suit. The warm up clothing will be transported to the finish line and will be waiting for you. For the actual race it is a good idea to buy a cheap long sleeve shirt that you can wear over your race clothing. Marathons usually start early in the morning when it is cool. You can start the race with two layers. When it warms up later in the race, you can discard the throw away shirt. The discarded shirts are collected by volunteers and are donated to a charitable organization.

Dressing for cold weather races are easier. Just wear the appropriate clothing for the weather conditions. You will probably wear the same clothing throughout the race.

Shoe Basics

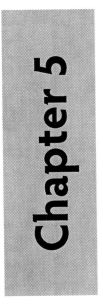

One of the great things about running is the low cost involved. There is no other sport or activity in the world that requires less equipment than running. All you need is a good pair of running shoes.

Today's running shoes are designed to provide comfort, correct bio-mechanical inefficiencies, prevent injuries and enhance performance. The best place to shop for shoes is at a running specialty store. Many of these retailers are small and as a result you may pay a little more for the shoes. How- 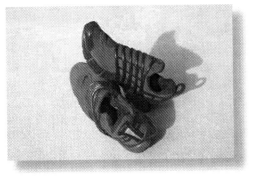 ever, the salespersons in a running store are usually running experts themselves and will be able to correctly advise you on the best shoe for your individual needs. If you buy at a large shoe or department store you should do your homework and determine which shoe is best for you. The salespersons in these large department stores usually know very little about running shoes or running biomechanics.

I have summarized the basics of running shoes below. If you are shopping without expert advice, follow the guidelines below and you should end up with a satisfactory purchase.

Shoe Construction

Shoes are made up of five components: the outer sole, the mid sole, the upper, the heel counter, and the slip lasting or board lasting. The **outer sole** is the bottom part of the shoe that contacts the ground. Shoes designed for 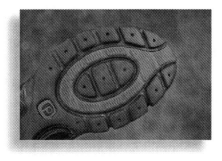 road running will have a variety of patterns on the bottom. Trail running shoes will have a large waffle or knobby pattern to provide better traction on dirt, grass and mud. The most important consideration of the outer sole is wear ability and traction. Some outer soles are softer than others. A hard outer sole will wear longer. A softer outer sole will provide a small amount of additional cushioning. This could be of benefit to a heavier runner. The softer material can also provide more traction on slick surfaces.

The **mid sole** is the part of the shoe just above the outer sole. The main function of the mid sole is to provide cushioning, stability, and flexibility. Earlier shoes had mid soles made of rubber. Most of today's shoes have some sort of combinations of vinyl compounds and air bladders or other lightweight shock absorbing materials. This has decreased the weight of shoes and increased their shock absorption abilities. Wear of the mid sole is the first sign that your shoes should be replaced. Most of the cushioning and shock absorption is located in the mid sole. As the mid sole wears, it becomes compressed and loses its ability to absorb the impact created when running. There is a rule of thumb that says to replace your shoes every 500 miles of running. You do not have to blindly follow this rule. Just check the cushioning of your mid soles frequently. Press on the mid sole at the heel, mid shoe and at the front of the shoe. If the mid sole feels compressed or feels like much of the cushioning is gone, you should replace the shoes.

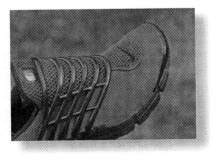

The **upper** is part of the shoe that wraps around your foot. This is usually made of a nylon material. The upper is either slip lasted or board lasted. **Slip lasting** means the nylon upper is tucked under and glued directly to the mid sole. This type of lasting provides more flexibility and is lighter in weight. In shoes that are **board lasted**, a board is placed over the tucked under portion of the upper. This type of shoe provides more stability and prevents pronation, which is the tendency for the foot to roll excessively to the inside. A board lasted shoe is best for a runner that pronates or supinates excessively. A slip lasted shoe will work well for a mechanically efficient runner.

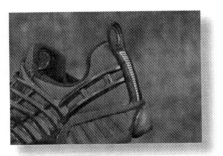

The **heel counter** is the stiff, molded portion of the shoe directly behind the heel. This feature will also reduce ankle pronation. The stiffer the heel counter the more protection the shoe has against pronation. Pinch the heel counter between your thumb and index finger. The harder it is to pinch the heel counter, the stronger the heel counter. A strong heel counter is better for runners that need a stable shoe.

Shoe Selection

The most important consideration in shoe selection is the biomechanics of your foot, the type of running you do, and your body type. When running or walking your foot will naturally roll to the inside or outside which is known as pronation and supination.

Pronation of the foot is a natural and normal motion during the footstrike. Pronation is simply the natural rolling inward of the foot. During a normal footstrike the foot rolls forward and to the inside, which provides cushioning. Many runners have excessive pronation, in which the foot rolls more to the inside than it should. If you do not know if you pronate or not, ask your sports physician, a running coach or a knowledgeable running specialty store salesperson

There is an easy way to determine if your feet pronate. It is the "wet foot" test. Take off your shoes and socks. Get your feet wet by stepping in water or wet grass. Now walk or run with your normal stride across some clean concrete. Take a close look at your footprints. If there is a print of your entire foot, including the arch, you are pronating. If your print shows the outside of your foot with a moon shaped cutout where your arch is, you do not pronate excessively.

to analyze your stride. They should be able to determine if you pronate excessively by watching your stride. If you can't determine if you pronate excessively or not, try purchasing a moderately priced running shoe with some stability features. After a few months of running, examine the bottom of the shoe. If it shows excessive wear on the inside, you probably are pronating excessively.

Supination is the excessive rolling of the foot to the outside. This is much more rare than pronation, but is still something you want to watch for.

Shoe Types

There are six primary types of shoes: stability shoes, lightweight trainers, cushioned shoes, racing flats, trail shoes and minimalist shoes.

Stability shoes are for runners that have moderate to severe pronation or supination problems. The stability features will add some weight, but will help prevent the injuries that the pronation can cause.

Lightweight trainers are made both with and without some stability features. Lightweight trainers without stability features are for daily running use and racing by runners with no stability problems. Trainers with some stability features are for daily use by runners with mild stability problems. These shoes are slightly heavier than the trainers without stability features are but lighter than the pure stability shoes.

The best place to shop for shoes is at a running speciality shop. Runners have special shoe needs. Sale people at running speciality shops are usually runners themselves and are more knowledgeable about running shoes. Many of these stores have a treadmill available for you to test run the shoes and also to check your running form.

Cushioned shoes are shoes with more cushioning materials than the other shoes. These shoes are popular among heavy runners or runners with joint problems. They are also used by efficient runners, with no mechanical problems, that desire a soft ride in a training shoe. These shoes are available with or without stability features.

Racing flats are ultralight shoes with little cushioning and few stability features. These shoes are usually worn only during races, since they do little to prevent injures and the wear ability is less than training shoes.

Trail shoes are more ruggedly built and have a heavier knobby outer sole to provide traction. These shoes usually have a lot of stability features because of the uneven terrain that is encountered on the trail.

Minimalist Shoes are shoes that mimic barefoot running as closely as possible. Running barefoot encourages proper running style and helps strengthen the muscles of your lower leg. These shoes have very little cushioning or support and are designed to allow your foot to work the way it was intended without the cast like effect of many standard running shoes. This type of shoe is becoming more popular, but you should adapt to these shoes gradually if your feet are not properly conditioned.

Shoe Fit

When you run, blood is pumped into your foot. As a result your feet and toes swell. If you don't have enough toe room, this can result in blisters and black toenails. You should have approximately one half inch of toe room. It is better to have a little more than a little less.

The heel should fit snugly, but not tight. The heel should not roll or move from side to side. When you bend your foot the heel should give only slightly.

Take the shoes for a test run around the store or around the parking lot before you purchase them. This is the only way to tell if they really fit and feel good. Make sure you are wearing the same kind of socks that you wear when you run. Just a slight difference in sock thickness will make a difference in how the shoe feels.

To test the mid sole for the amount of its stability, hold the shoe with the heel in your right hand and the forefoot in your left hand. Twist the shoe like a dish rag. If the shoe twists easily, it has less stability. If it is harder to twist, it has more stability. The more stable shoes are best for motion control or for runners that pronate excessively.

Other Considerations

Do not buy a shoe that is marginally small. You foot will swell a bit when you run. So, if the shoe is already small, it will become very uncomfortable when you run. You should be able to fit the width of your finger in between your longest toe and the front of the shoe.

Do not buy a shoe because of looks. While it is certainly nice to wear a good looking shoe, the important thing is fit, comfort and using the shoe that is appropriate for your running style. Try out a lot of shoes. There are a lot of different models and styles out there. Each individual shoe will feel and fit a bit differently. First, be sure you're buying the shoe that is right for your running mechanics. Second, from the available shoe for your running style, pick the shoe that is most comfortable. Third, from the shoes you have picked out, choose the one that you feel looks the best.

If this is your first pair of running shoes, consider buying a moderately priced pair. Run with them for a while and see how they perform. If they turn out to be the right type of shoe, you can spend more on your next pair. If they do not work out well, you can try a different type of shoe next time.

Aches and Pains

Injuries are a common occurrence in any athletic activity and running is no exception. The typical experienced runner takes around 180 strides each minute. During a 30 minute run that is 5,400 strides. During a 4 hour marathon you would take a whopping 43,200 strides! During each stride you will place between 1.5 and 4 times your body weight on your feet, depending upon how efficiently you run and how fast you are going. Taking an average of 2 times body weight a 150 pound runner would place almost 13 million pounds of stress on their feet and legs during a 4 hour marathon!

Every runner is hobbled by an injury from time to time. Contrary to popular opinion, intense or fast running is not the cause of most running injuries. Most running injuries are causes by overuse or overtraining. In other words if you try to do too much, too soon, you are at a greater risk of suffering from an

Injuries are an unavoidable risk in running. You can avoid most common running injuries through proper training and running form

injury. That's why beginning runners need to gradually increase their training mileage. As a new runner, if you were to go out and try to run 5 miles on your very first workout, you would certainly be sore the next day and could even end up with muscle or joint injuries. Even experienced runners need to be careful when training. They must make all increases in mileage or intensity gradually. They also should include periods of rest and recovery in their training programs in order to avoid overtraining problems such as chronic fatigue, soreness, illness, frequent injuries and burnout. Overuse and overtraining are the most common causes of injuries but they do not stand alone. Poor running form, muscle weakness, muscle tightness, muscle imbalance, improper shoes and choice of running surface all contribute to running injuries.

Avoiding Injuries

It is very difficult to completely avoid all running injuries, but they are something that proper training techniques will help avoid. If you run efficiently and avoid training errors you will minimize your chances of becoming injured. Here are some tips to help keep away those bothersome aches and pains.

Stretching

Stretching provides three benefits to you as a runner. It reduces your risk of injury; decreases muscle soreness and improves performance. There are six basic stretching techniques: static, passive, dynamic, ballistic, proprioceptive neuromuscular facilitation (PNF) and active isolated (AI).

•   **Static stretching** - This is the most commonly used technique. A stretch position is gently assumed and held for 20 to 60 seconds. There is no bouncing or rapid movement. Do not stretch to the point of pain. You should feel a slight pull, but no discomfort. Keep all joints in alignment.

Do not twist joints into unnatural positions. The stretch should be felt in the belly of the muscle and not in the joints. This type of stretch works best after your workout rather than before.

- **Passive stretching** - This basic technique is the same as static stretching. The muscles are kept relaxed and a gentle stretch is maintained for 20 to 60 seconds. The difference with a passive stretch is that a helper actually provides the force of the stretch. In a static stretch, you get your body into position and supply the force for the stretch with other muscle groups and using body weight. With passive stretching you relax your entire body, while a helper provides the force to stretch your muscles. The same rules apply here. There should be no bouncing or rapid movement. Do not stretch to the point of pain.

- **Dynamic stretching** - A current popular buzzword among athletes is functional training. That basically means training that mimics the activity you are training for. Dynamic stretching could be also be called functional stretching. A dynamic stretch is one in which your limbs are moving through their full range of motion. For example, walking with high knees is a dynamic flexibility exercise that stretches your glutes, quadriceps and lower back. These stretching exercises are best performed after a warm up and before you begin your activity. Note that these stretches are often re-

Recent studies have proven what running coaches have known for years. Excessive stretching does little to prevent injury and can actually decrease your running performance. The best stretching routine uses dynamic stretching before your workout and gentle static stretching after your run. The dynamic stretches prepare your muscles for your workout while the post-run static stretching helps keep your muscles healthy and flexible.

ferred to as warm up drills rather than actual stretches. The term "drills" may be a more accurate description because of the active, functional nature of dynamic exercises.

• **Ballistic stretching** is a rapid bouncing up and down. This type of stretching applies more than twice the tension as a passive or ballistic stretch. Ballistic stretching is appropriate only for a very limited number of athletes. The rapid bouncing can cause more damage than flexibility. It can be used for some highly conditioned athletes that need to prepare for a volatile, high-speed activity. It is not an appropriate technique for a beginning runner.

• **Proprioceptive neuromuscular facilitation (PNF)** was originally developed by physical therapists for rehabilitation purposes. This type of stretch is accomplished by maximally contracting the muscle to be stretched for 5 to 10 seconds. This is followed by a slow passive stretch. This is repeated several times. By contracting the muscle and then stretching, you overcome a tendency for the muscle to resist the stretch, which results in a higher degree of flexibility.

• **Active isolated (AI) stretching** is the latest development is flexibility. AI stretching involves contracting the opposing muscle while the target muscle is stretched. The theory is that as one muscle is contracted, the opposing muscle will relax. An example of opposing muscles are the hamstrings on the back of the thigh and the quadriceps muscles on the front of the thigh. By contracting the quadriceps as you stretch the hamstrings, the hamstrings will relax to a greater degree, resulting in a better stretch. Many dynamic stretches are a form of AI stretching.

Recommendations

The recommended methods are dynamic stretching or drills before your training run and either static or AI stretching after your workout. Ballistic stretching has been shown to be a high-risk type of stretch. Studies show that AI stretching provides more flexibility than either passive or static stretching. However, all of the stretches, with the exception of ballistic stretching, are appropriate for beginning runners. You should stay away from ballistic stretching, which is reserved for more highly trained athletes.

Strength Training

Many injuries can be prevented by strength training. Strong and flexible muscles will be less prone to pulling and straining. Strong muscles will provide support to joints and connective tissue. This is especially true for the knee and shoulder joints, which are biomechanically loose and weak joints. A properly designed strength training program will also help correct muscle imbalances that can contribute to the cause of injury. An example of muscle imbalances are the hamstrings on the back of your upper leg and the quadriceps muscles on the front of your upper legs. In runners, the hamstrings tend to get strong and tight. The quadriceps muscles are weaker and less developed. This results in an imbalance that can cause hip or back injuries and pain. Strengthening the quadriceps muscles with strength training will correct and prevent this imbalance.

A well designed strength training program will help you avoid injury, decrease your body fat and improve your overall level of fitness

If you are new to strength training, be sure to start slow and easy. Don't lift heavy weights until you are familiar with proper weight lifting procedures and have built up a strong base. Educate your self on proper weight lifting techniques or set an appointment with a personal trainer to get the proper instruction. Poor weight lifting technique can result in injury.

Do not begin running or any exercise program with high intensity work. You must let your body gradually adapt to the new stresses being put on it. Starting an exercise program at too high of a level is not only a cause of many injuries, but is one of the top causes of abandonment of an exercise program. By starting slowly you will allow your muscles and connective tissues to grow stronger so they can support the higher intensity exercise that will follow.

Be sure to give your body plenty of rest. The rest should come daily by getting plenty of sleep and weekly by incorporating rest days into your program. Muscles and connective tissue require consistent periods of rest to recover. The muscles, which become broken down during periods of intense exercise, rebuild and become stronger during rest periods. Your body will let you know if you are not getting enough rest. You may feel sluggish and tired. You may have muscle and joint pain. Listen to your body. If you think you need rest, take a day off.

Treating Injuries

There will probably be times when you become injured despite taking every precaution. Here are some treatment tips for common injuries. This does not substitute for advice of a doctor. You should always consult with your sports physician when you become injured.

RICE

The initial and most important level of self treatment for most sports injuries is referred to by the acronym RICE. This stands for rest, ice, compression and elevation. RICE should be performed as soon as possible after an injury happens. Fast treatment can make the difference between days and weeks of recovery time.

- **Rest** - The first step in treating any injury is to stop the activity. During the first 24 to 48 hours, complete rest is usually required. Later in your recovery, it is better to include some light activity so that you can avoid muscle atrophy, stiffness and reduced range of motion. You should continue with complete rest or light activity until you can perform your activity pain free.

- **Ice** - Icing or cooling your injury will decrease swelling, bleeding and pain. You should apply ice to the injured area for approximately 20 minutes, 3 to 4 times a day. A good way to do this is to use a bag of frozen peas. Just keep them in your freezer and they are ready to go when you need them. The peas will form nicely around your knee, ankle, elbow and most any other injured body part. If you use a bag of ice, cover your injured area with a wet towel and apply the bag of ice over the towel. Continue this ice therapy until the swelling and pain are gone.

- **Compression** - Application of compression, usually through the use of an elastic wrap, will help reduce swelling by forcing fluid back into the circulatory system of the body. Wrap the injured area firmly, but not so tight as to cut off circulation. Start the wrap a couple of inches above the injury and continue a couple inches below the injured area.

- **Elevation** - Gravity tends to pull fluids and blood towards your injury. This is one of the causes of swelling and pain. Elevation of the injured part of your body will assist in returning fluids to the system. Try to keep your injured area above the level of your heart.

Severe or Chronic Injuries

If you are suffering from a severe injury, a chronic injury or an injury that will not heal, you should see a physician. It is best to consult with a physician that specializes in sports medicine. If you can find one that is also a runner, it would be ideal. Sports doctors will have the specialized knowledge and experience necessary to properly deal with running injuries.

Many times a doctor that is not a sports specialist or is not active in sports, will tell you to quit running if you get injured. In the vast majority of cases, this is bad advice. Any injury that is caused by running has a cause that can be corrected. A sports specialist and fellow runner will understand this and will help you find a solution. The benefits that you gain from running, far outweigh the inconvenience of occasional injury. If your doctor tells you that you must quit running, get a second opinion from a sports specialist. Podiatrists (foot doctors), chiropractors and physical therapists are other sources of assistance with injuries.

Common Running Injuries

Here are some descriptions of common running injuries and some suggestions for self treatment. This information is provided for educational purposes only and is not a substitute for proper medical advise. Self-diagnosis of injuries is not recommended. See your doctor for diagnosis and treatment of all injuries.

Shin Splints

Shin splints have become a catchall phrase for an aching pain on the front of the lower leg. This generic term is used to describe several different conditions. The most common is a sprain or tear of the posterior tibial muscle, which is located at the back of your lower leg bone. Other conditions include an inflammation of the covering of the bone, a stress fracture of the tibia and anterior compartment syndrome, which is a restriction of the blood flow to the muscles at the front of the lower leg. All of the conditions are caused by overuse or intense exercise before the muscles are properly conditioned. Strengthening and stretching of the muscles on the front of the lower leg will help prevent this injury.

A true shin splint is a tearing of the muscle fiber where it attaches to the tibia. This causes a dull pain on the inside part of the front of the lower leg bone. Shin splints should be treated with rest, ice and an anti-inflammatory such as aspirin. This is a very common running injury. Running downhill or running on hard surfaces such as concrete will increase the chances of having this injury. Stretching the front of the lower leg by "sitting" on your feet, with your feet sole up and extended behind you and leaning backwards will help prevent shin splints. If you do this stretch, be sure your feet are directly under you legs, not out to the side.

• **Tibial periostitis** or swelling of the covering of the bone is recognized by touch. The tender area will be just under the skin, above the bone on the front of the lower leg. The pain will begin about three inches above the ankle. This should be treated with rest, ice and an anti-inflammatory such as aspirin. If the pain does not subside in a few days, see your doctor.

• **Anterior compartment syndrome** involves the muscles on the outside part of the front of your lower leg. These muscles are surrounded by a box of fascial covering. As the muscles are exercised they swell with blood. The surrounding box pushes back against the swelling and constricts the blood flow to the muscles, causing pain. Pain caused by this injury will be in the muscles on the outside part of the front of the lower leg. This condition should be treated with rest, ice and an anti-inflammatory. Severe and chronic cases may require minor surgery to relieve the pressure. You should see your doctor if you suspect this injury. If you feel any numbness in your foot or lower leg, see your doctor immediately. Severe swelling can cause circulation to be diminished, which can be a serious condition.

• **Tibial stress fracture** is a small crack in the lower leg bone. The pain from a stress fracture will be dull and aching at first; and will be centered in one small spot. Later the pain will become severe and will not allow exercise.

A sports physician should diagnose the stress fracture. It is impossible to self-diagnose a stress fracture. Treatment will require rest for four to six weeks. A cast is usually not required.

Shin splints in runners are often caused by landing heavily on your heel. That is why downhill running contributes to the occurrence of this injury. When you land on your heel, the muscles on the front of your lower leg activate in an attempt to keep the front of your foot from "slapping" hard on the ground. That repeated stress can cause shin splints. Landing under your center of gravity on the ball of your foot or flat footed will help you avoid this injury.

Runner's Knee

Runner's knee is a very common injury among female runners because of the "Q-angle." Your Q-angle is determined by the angle created by a line traveling from your hip joint to your knee joint. Wider hips result in a larger Q-angle. A larger Q-angle results in more stress on your knee joint. Since women typically have wider hips than men it follows that this injury is more common among women. Other contributing factors include knock knees and excessive pronation (rolling inward) of the foot.

Runner's knee is the most common injury among runners. Surveys have shown that around 30 percent of the more than 15 million joggers in America suffer from runner's knee. Runner's knee is an overuse injury. The pain is located around the knee, usually on the outside part of the kneecap. Multiple areas of tearing in the sleeve surrounding the knee or a mis-tracking knee cap cause the pain.

The pain from runner's knee usually begins with mild discomfort and progresses to a major ache or sharp stabbing pain. The pain is not localized and is hard to pinpoint. The cause of runner's knee is usually inappropriate shoes or biomechanical inefficiency in the foot. It can also be caused by weak quadriceps muscles, which results in the knee cap tending to mis-track. You may need shoes that provide more stability or special orthotics. Consult with your sports physician, who will be able to analyze your stride and your shoes. Runner's knee should be treated with rest, ice and anti-inflammatory medicines such as aspirin.

Chondromalacia

Chondromalacia is wear and tear on the back of the kneecap. The pain caused by chondromalacia is located directly behind the kneecap. The pain may intensify with long periods of sitting. When you bend your knee while sitting you may hear a grinding sound or feel a grinding sensation. Chondromalacia is treated with rest and anti-inflammatory medicine. Strengthening of the quadriceps muscles on the front of the thigh may help this condition.

Plantar Fasciitis

Plantar fasciitis is a tear in the arch ligament on the bottom of the foot. This is the most common heel injury in runners. The pain experienced with this injury is located just under the front part of the heel bone. The pain is usually worse in the morning. Plantar fasciitis should be treated with rest, ice and anti-inflammatory medicine such as aspirin. If you have this injury you may need an orthotic in your shoe to support the arch. A good way to ice this injury is by freezing water in paper cups. You can roll the bottom of your foot over the iced cups.

Achilles Tendinitis

The Achilles tendon is the largest tendon in the body. It connects your calf muscles to the heel bone. This tendon is used constantly when running and jumping. Achilles tendinitis is an inflammation of this tendon. There is a sheath surrounding the tendon. The lining of this sheath becomes inflamed which restricts movement and causes pain. During the early stages of this injury the tendon will be painful when you squeeze it. You may not feel pain when you run in the early stages. By checking your Achilles tendon occasionally, you may be able to avoid a more severe Achilles injury.

In addition to the pain, you may hear or feel a grinding sensation when the tendon is moved. This injury should be treated with RICE. Rest for at least one week. Then begin a stretching and strengthening program. If the tendon responds positively to the treatment, you may slowly resume your running program. If the pain remains, you should consult your sports physician.

Blisters

Blisters are caused by friction. They most commonly occur on the feet and are caused by shoes that are too tight or skin that has not been toughened to the stresses of running. Running for an extended time in wet shoes or socks can also cause these annoying and painful injuries. Blisters will usually heal on their own. If you tend to get blisters, try covering the sensitive areas with mole skin or a similar product that will protect the area.

Side Stitch

A side stitch or side ache is not technically an injury. But it can be more disabling than many real injuries. Once, during an important cross-country competition, I suffered a side stitch so severe that I had to run doubled over. My coach appeared and reminded me that no one has ever died from a side stitch and told me to straighten up. After shooting him my most poisonous glare, I gamely continued on. Needless to say, his unappreciated advice did little to make me feel better. However, he was right. A side stitch is a painful condition, but is not medically dangerous unless it is a continuous problem. If you have a frequent or continuous pain in your side, see your doctor.

Side stitches have been a bit of a mystery. Researchers have not been able to pin down the exact cause of the cramps. The latest research has narrowed it down to two possible causes. One possible cause in centered around the ligaments that attach your stomach to your diaphragm. The movements of running causes a bouncing movement of your stomach which pulls on these ligaments. This causes a pain in your diaphragm. This would explain why stitches are more common when you run after eating or drinking a large amount. Another possible cause is related to blood flow in the trunk of your body. When you run, blood is diverted from the diaphragm to the working muscles of the legs. This results in the diaphragm being starved for oxygen, causing the cramp.

Nearly all runners struggle with the occasional side stitch. They are more common among beginning runners. As your fitness level increases you will have fewer problems with these annoying pains

A 1999 study published in Medicine & Science in Sports and Medicine[1], investigated both of these theories. The study showed that the most likely cause is the ligament theory. With this in mind, the following tips should help you avoid future side stitches.

• Do not run until 3 hours after a large meal. You will want your stomach to be mostly emptied before you start to run.

• Drink small amounts of fluid frequently, rather than a large amount more infrequently.

• Perform abdominal crunches daily. The tighter and stronger abdominal muscles will help support the stomach and diaphragm.

---

1   Medicine & Science in Sports & Exercise, 31(8):1169-1175 August 1999

If you get a stitch, contract your abdominal muscles to support your stomach. Breath with your belly. You should feel your belly move in and out as you breath, this will also help stabilize your stomach. Place pressure directly on the point of the pain with your fingers or the heel of your palm.

Eating and Drinking

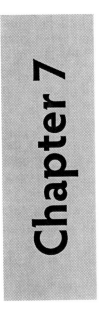

A s a runner and athlete, you will need to change the way you look at food. For a runner, food is not just the main course of a social event or a way to satisfy a hunger. Food is fuel. Food is energy. Food contains the building blocks of your muscles. It is what allows a runner to train and perform at peak efficiency.

Some people believe that runners can eat whatever they want to because they just burn it off. While running does burn a lot of calories, that statement is completely wrong. A runner must eat a sufficient amount of the right foods in order to keep their body operating at its highest level. A runner must eat for both top performance and for disease prevention.

Many runners are tempted to live on a diet of those tasty, high fat, junk foods that we have grown to love. Because of the charged up metabolism and high calorie burn that runners enjoy, a poor diet probably won't show up as weight gain. But, as a runner, you must consider the impact on long term health and on running performance. The health effects of a poor diet may not show up for many years, but it will eventually rear its ugly head.

You also must put the proper fuel in your body for top performance. A poor diet can result in lower endurance levels, low levels of speed and strength, sluggishness, lack of motivation and depression. Problems with the diet will also contribute to the occurrence of colds and other illnesses.

Types of Nutrients

Food is more than something to satisfy your appetite. Food is fuel for your body. There are many kinds of foods, but each food is composed of some sort of mix of six different types of nutrients. Each type of nutrient has a specific purpose and meets a specific need that your body has. The six nutrients are: water, carbohydrates, protein, fat, vitamins and minerals.

Water

Yes, water is a nutrient. Not only is it a nutrient, it is the most important nutrient. In fact, your body is approximately 55 to 60 percent water. Your body uses water 24 hours a day. A by-product of the energy production in your body is heat. Water regulates your body temperature by dissipating that heat. Water also carries nutrients to the cells in your body. Water does not produce energy.

Water is an especially crucial nutrient for runners. Insufficient water will result in dehydration and reduced blood volume. Your blood volume increases as you become fitter. The higher blood volume results in improved oxygen delivery to your working muscles. When your blood volume decreases because of inadequate water, your performance suffers. Blood volume is also a critical factor in preventing heat related disorders.

You lose water through the production of energy and through your body's efforts to keep cool, more simply called sweating. The energy production processes in your body generate a tremendous amount of heat. Your body dissipates that heat by producing sweat. The sweat evaporates and cools your body. During an hour of running, you will lose more that 2 quarts of water, through sweating.

Most runners fall short of replacing the lost water. As your body dehydrates, your blood thickens and the delivery of oxygen to your muscles slows. As a result, your pace slows and you begin to feel fatigued.

Make sure you stay well hydrated at all times. Do not wait until you feel thirsty to drink. Your feelings of thirst will lag behind your hydration levels. If you wait until you feel thirsty, you are already dehydrated. When you are running try to drink at least a cup of water every 15 minutes.

Carbohydrates

Carbohydrates are the primary source of energy for your body. Carbohydrates power every system in your body, including your brain, heart, muscles and internal organs.

Carbohydrates can be simple (table sugar, corn syrup) or complex (whole grain). Simple carbohydrates enter your bloodstream very quickly. That is why you get a sugar high when you eat candy. The sudden rush of glucose into your bloodstream gives you that quick burst of energy. When the glucose enters the bloodstream your brain sends a signal to release insulin into your blood. Insulin helps your cells absorb the blood glucose. The resulting rapid absorption of glucose causes the tired feeling you get shortly after a sugar high. Complex carbohydrates are processed and used more slowly. They do not give your body the roller coaster ride of high and low energy that a simple carbohydrate will.

Protein

Protein is like the brick and mortar of your body. It is the building blocks that provide the structure for the tissues of your body. Proteins are also used to transport essential elements in your blood stream.

Some proteins are working proteins and some are structural. Structural proteins make up your muscles, ligaments, tendons, nails and hair. Working proteins include anti-bodies, enzymes, transports, hormones and oxygen carriers. It is the structure of proteins that allow them to carry out so many tasks. Proteins are composed of amino acids. There are 20 amino acids. A protein could contain all 20 amino acids. The number and configuration of these amino acids, determines the job of each protein.

Your body can manufacture about half of the 20 amino acids, using other nutrients in your body. The other half must be provided in your diet. These are called essential amino acids. Since your body must have the proteins that essential amino acids provide, you must eat foods that supply these amino acids on a daily basis.

Fats

The omega-3 fatty acids found in cold water fish help protect your body from heart disease, hypertension, arthritis and cancer. If you prefer not to eat fish there are a number of omega-3 supplements available that are also beneficial

Fats are our storehouses of energy. When we have excess nutrients in our body, some of it is stored as fat. The primary purpose of fat is energy production. Fat is our body's most powerful form of energy. One gram of fat supplies 9 calories of energy to the body. In comparison, carbohydrates and protein provide only 4 calories of energy per gram.

The energy potential of fat is critical in successfully completing a marathon. You cannot store enough carbohydrates in your body to energize your muscles through 26.2 miles of running without drawing upon the vast stores of energy that is contained in your fat reservoirs.

When a marathon runner hits the dreaded "wall", they have usually depleted their muscles of glycogen, the storage form of carbohydrates. Successfully running a marathon, without smashing into the wall, depends upon your body using fat to produce much of the energy required to fuel your running, while sparing your valuable stores of carbohydrates.

There are two main types of fats – saturated and unsaturated. Animal fats (meat, butter, lard) are usually saturated fats and contribute to heart disease and cancer. Vegetable fats (olive oil, corn oil) are generally unsaturated fats and are less harmful. Some fats have been found to be helpful in preventing some cancers and heart disease. These fats called omega-3 fatty acids are found in some fish, especially cold-water fish. Most of us eat too much fat. Most experts say that we should cut back on fats, but the agreements end there. Some think that a diet that contains around 30% fat is the best way to go, while others believe that it should be cut to as low as 10%.

Vitamins

Vitamins are essential for the regulation of many of the functions of your body. Most vitamins cannot be manufactured by your body and must be obtained from your diet or from supplements. Vitamins do not produce energy but they do play an important role in making possible the processes by which other nutrients are digested, absorbed and utilized.

Vitamins are either fat soluble or water soluble. Fat soluble vitamins can be stored in fat and because of that storablility, can build up to toxic levels. Water soluble vitamins are not stored in tissues. Any excess water soluble vitamin is excreted in the urine and are less likely to cause any toxicity issues.

The fat soluble vitamins are A, D, E and K. Water soluble vitamins are B, C, thiamin, riboflavin, niacin, folate B_{12}, B_6, biotin and pantothenic acid. B_6 can build up to toxic levels even though it is a water soluble vitamin.

Vitamins - Functions and Food Sources

Vitamin	What It Does	Where You Get It	What You Need To Know
A	Vision, immune system, skin & bone growth	Sweet potato, carrot, spinach, tomatoes, milk, whole wheat bread	Excess vitamin A can be toxic. Beta carotene is a non-toxic source
D	Immune system, bone growth, absorption of calcium	Sunlight, fortified milk, liver	The most potentially toxic of all vitamins.
E	Anti-oxidant	Green leafy vegetables, whole grain products, nuts, seeds	Least toxic of the fat soluble vitamins
K	Blood clotting, bone formation	Green leafy vegetables, milk	
Thiamin	Energy metabolism, nervous system function	All nutritious foods, whole grains, nuts	Also called vitamin B1
Riboflavin	Energy metabolism, vision, skin health	Milk, yogurt, whole grains, green leafy vegetables, enriched cereals	Also known as vitamin B2
Niacin	Energy metabolism, nervous system function, skin health	Milk, eggs, poultry, fish, whole grain, enriched cereals	Also called nicotinic acid
B6	Helps make red blood cells, amino and fatty acid metabolism	Green leafy vegetables, meats, fish, poultry, legumes fruits, whole grains	Large doses can be dangerous
Folate	New cell synthesis	Green leafy vegetables, legumes, seeds	Also known as folic acid, vulnerable to interactions with medications
B12	New cell synthesis, maintains nerve cells	Meat, fish, poultry, eggs, milk, cheese	Works closely with folate

Vitamins - Functions and Food Sources

Vitamin	What It Does	Where You Get It	What You Need To Know
Panothenic Acid	Energy metabolism	All nutritious foods	Stimulates growth
Biotin	Energy metabolism, amino and fatty acid metabolism, glyocgen synthesis	All nutritious foods	Deficiencies are rare
C	Strengthens blood vessels, antioxidant, amino acid metabolism, strengthens immune system, helps absorb iron	Citrus fruits, dark green vegetables, strawberries, peppers, tomatoes	Also called ascorbic acid

Minerals

Minerals are compounds, obtained from your diet, that combine in several ways to form the structures of your body. For instance, calcium is a mineral that is crucial in the formation and maintenance of your bones. Minerals also help regulate body functions. Minerals do not produce energy. The following table shows the function of common minerals and what they do for you.

Minerals - Functions and Food Sources

Mineral	What It Does	Where You Get It	What You Need To Know
Calcium	Bone and tooth growth and health. Helps with muscle contraction and relaxation	Milk and milk products, tofu, greens, legumes	The most important mineral for bone health. Also important for nerve transmission
Phosphorus	Energy transfer. Growth of cells	Milk, beans, meats, fish	The second most abundant mineral in the body
Magnesium	Bone growth, enzyme activity and muscle contraction	Whole grains, nuts, legumes, dark green leafy vegetables	Unprocessed foods are the best source
Sodium	Maintains fluid balance, essential for muscle contraction and nerve transmission	Salt, soy sauce, processed foods	Abundantly available in nearly all of today's foods
Chloride	Digestion	Salt, sour sauce, processed foods	
Potassium	Maintains fluid & electrolyte balance, muscle contractions, nerve transmission	Whole foods, milk, meats, fruits, vegetables, grains, legumes	Also critical in maintain the heartbeat.
Iodine	Helps regulate growth and metabolic rate	Iodized salt, seafood	Non-iodized sea salt is not a good source
Iron	Part of the oxygen carrying hemoglobin in the blood cells	Red meat, fish, poultry, eggs, legumes, dried fruit	Iron is toxic in large amounts
Zinc	Assists enzymes	Foods containing protein	

Minerals - Functions and Food Sources			
Mineral	What It Does	Where You Get It	What You Need To Know
Selenium	Helps break down chemicals that harm cells	Seafoods, meats, grains	Assists vitamin E as an anti-oxidant

Reading Food Labels

Thanks to the Nutrition Labeling and Education Act of 1990 (NLEA), we can get all the nutritional information that we need, right on the label of most foods. Most foods are required to provide this labeling. The foods that are exempt from this rule are:

• Food served for immediate consumption (airline, mall cookies)

• Ready to eat food prepared on site (bakery, deli, candy store)

• Food shipped in bulk.

• Medical foods used to meet needs of patients with certain diseases.

• Plain coffee and tea or other foods that have little or no nutritional value.

Nutritional Facts Label

The "Nutrition Facts" panel on the label contains information that is very useful in planning your daily meals. The first section tells you the serving

Nutrition Facts
Serving Size 1 cup (228g)
Servings Per Container 2

Amount Per Serving
Calories 260   Calories from Fat 120

                                          % Daily Value*
Total Fat 13g   **20%**
   Saturated Fat 5g   **25%**
   Trans Fat 2g
Cholesterol 30mg   **10%**
Sodium 660mg   **28%**
Total Carbohydrate 31g   **10%**
   Dietary Fiber 0g   **0%**
   Sugars 5g
Protein 5g

Vitamin A 4%   •   Vitamin C 2%
Calcium 15%   •   Iron 4%

* Percent Daily Values are based on a 2,000 calorie diet. Your Daily Values may be higher or lower depending on your calorie needs:

	Calories	2,000	2,500
Total Fat	Less than	65g	80g
Sat Fat	Less than	20g	25g
Cholesterol	Less than	300mg	300mg
Sodium	Less than	2,400mg	2,400mg
Total Carbohydrate		300g	375g
Dietary Fiber		25g	30g

Calories per gram:
Fat 9   •   Carbohydrate 4   •   Protein 4

size and number of servings in the package. This is the starting point for determining the exact number of calories and nutrients in the food. The next section shows the calories per serving and the number of fat calories per serving, which is the most important information for anyone that is trying to lose weight. The other areas of the label will give you the nutritional content of the food, such as total fat, saturated fats, trans fats, cholesterol, sodium, carbohydrates, dietary fiber, sugars and protein. It will also tell you the some of the vitamins contained in the food. The bottom section gives you a breakdown of the percentage of daily values you should be getting in a typical healthy diet.

Daily Values

Daily values are designed to reflect the recommended daily allowance (RDA) of the nutrients on the food label. If the daily value is 5%, it means that one serving provides 5% of the RDA for that nutrient. Fats, cholesterol and sodium are expressed as maximum amounts you should have for a healthy diet. Using the sample table as an example, your sodium intake should be less than 2,400 mg.

Ingredient List

When you know how to read an ingredient list you have the key to selecting the healthiest food choice. The first ingredient listed is the one that is of the greatest quantity by weight. Look at any of the most popular powdered drink mixes. You will see that sugar is the first listed ingredient. You can now tell that the product is predominately sugar.

There are some things that you will want to be careful with. Look at some of the wheat breads. Many will show wheat flour as the first ingredient. Seeing this, you may think you are getting whole wheat bread. You are not. White flour is also wheat flour. The first ingredient in whole wheat bread will say whole-wheat flour or whole grain. Also remember that corn syrup, honey, dextrose, fructose and sucrose are all different versions of sugar.

Nutrient Content Claims

Many products make claims such as "fat free", "lean" or "low fat". There are regulations that define what terms may be used to describe the level of nutrients in foods. Here are the terms and their requirements:

• **Free** – This means a product that contains no amount of or an insignificant amount of fat, saturated fat, cholesterol, sodium, sugars or calories. Fat free means less than 0.5 grams per serving. Calorie free means less than 5 calories per serving.

• **Low** – This means foods that can be eaten frequently without exceeding guidelines for fat, saturated fat, cholesterol, sodium or calories.

• **Lean and extra lean** – These terms describe the fat content of meat, fish and poultry. Lean means less than 10 grams of fat, 4.5 grams or less of saturated fat and less than 95 mg of cholesterol per 100 grams. Extra lean means less than 5 grams of fat, less than 2 grams of saturated fat and less than 95 mg of cholesterol per 100 grams.

• **High** – This describes a food that contains 20 percent or more of the Daily Value for a nutrient.

• **Good Source** – This means a food that contains 10 to 19 percent of the Daily Value of a nutrient.

• **Reduced** – This means a food that has been altered to contain at least 25 percent less of a nutrient or calories than the normal version of the food.

• **Less** – This is similar to reduced except the food may or may not be altered.

• **Light** – This describes a food that has been altered to contain 1/3 fewer calories or ½ of the fat of the normal unaltered food.

- **More** – This means that the food contains at least 10 percent more of the Daily Value than the referenced food.

- **Healthy** – In order for a food to be described as "Healthy" it must be low in fat and saturated fat and contain limited amounts of cholesterol and sodium. It must contain at least 10 percent more of vitamins C or A, iron, calcium, protein or fiber. Sodium content cannot exceed 360 mg per serving.

- **Fresh** – The term fresh can only be used when the food is raw, never frozen or heated and contains no preservatives. Fresh frozen can be used if the food is quickly frozen while fresh. Terms such as fresh milk or freshly baked bread are not a part of this regulation.

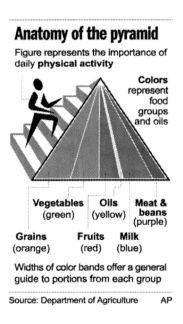

Anatomy of the pyramid

Figure represents the importance of daily **physical activity**

Colors represent food groups and oils

Vegetables (green)   Oils (yellow)   Meat & beans (purple)

Grains (orange)   Fruits (red)   Milk (blue)

Widths of color bands offer a general guide to portions from each group

Source: Department of Agriculture   AP

The Food Pyramid

The most commonly used guide for food choices is the food guide pyramid. In 2005, the USDA released a new version of the food pyramid. The new pyramid follows the 2005 U.S. Dietary Guidelines which emphasize the importance of whole grains, vegetables, fruits and healthful fats, while limiting the consumption of sugar, saturated fats and trans fats.

The food pyramid makes dietary recommendations that are specific to specific age and sex group categories.

Keep in mind that the food pyramid recommendations are very general in nature. Your specific caloric and nutrient needs depend upon your activity level, your goals and your current level of health and fitness. There is no one answer to the question of what and how much you should be eating, but the food pyramid is a good starting point and does offer good suggestions for overall eating patterns.

The new food pyramid has come under some criticism from some parts of nutritional profession. The two most common criticisms of the new version are:

• The new pyramid is primarily web based and is therefore hard to use in the print version.

• The old pyramid made more specific recommendations as far as food choices and portion sizes.

The old food pyramid made the following recommendations:

• Bread, cereal and other grains - 6 to 11 servings.

• Fruit – 2 to 4 servings.

• Vegetables – 3 to 5 servings.

• Milk, yogurt and cheese – 2 to 3 servings.

• Meat, poultry, fish, eggs, beans, nuts – 2 to 3 servings.

• Fats, oils and sweets – Use sparingly.

So now that you know how many servings to eat, you still don't know how much to eat! Below is a guide that will show you how much food actually makes up a serving.

Bread, cereal and other grains

These foods provide complex carbohydrates, fiber and many vitamins and nutrients including: riboflavin, thiamin, iron, protein and niacin. One serving size equals: 1 slice of bread, ½ bagel, ½ bun, 1 cup of dry cereal, ½ cup of cooked cereal, ½ cup of rice, ½ cup of pasta, 1 small roll or muffin, 2 large crackers. One half cup is about the size of your computer mouse.

Fruits

Fruits contribute vitamin C, vitamin A, fiber and potassium as well as a number of vitamins. One serving of fruit equals: 1 medium fruit such as an apple, banana or orange, ½ large fruit such as a grapefruit, 1 melon wedge, ½ cup of berries, ¾ cup of fruit juice, ½ cup of canned fruit, ¼ cup of dried fruit.

Vegetables

Vegetables contribute vitamin C, vitamin A, folate, potassium, magnesium, fiber and a number of other vitamins and minerals. One serving equals: ½ cup of raw or cooked vegetables, ¾ cup of vegetable juice, and 1 cup of raw leafy vegetables. One cup is about the size of a baseball.

Milk, yogurt and cheese

These foods contribute protein, calcium, riboflavin, vitamin B, vitamin D and vitamin A. One serving equals: 1 cup of milk, 1 cup of yogurt, 1 and ½ oz. of cheese.

Meat, poultry, fish, eggs, beans and nuts

These foods provide protein, vitamin B, zinc, magnesium, iron, niacin and thiamin. One serving equals: 2 to 3 oz. of lean meat (about the size of a deck of standard playing cards), poultry or fish, 1 egg, ½ cup of cooked beans, 2 Tbs of peanut butter.

Fats, oils and sweets

These foods contribute very few nutrients and no serving recommendations have been suggested.

THE GLYCEMIC INDEX

Diets that decrease and in some cases eliminate carbohydrates have become extremely popular in the past couple of years. Just look in the diet section of your local bookstore. It is filled with dozens of books telling you that carbohydrates are the greatest nutrition evil of our time.

Carbohydrates are not evil. They are necessary for energy production and general health. Carbohydrates supply the energy needed to keep your heart, brain and vital organs operating. However, these types of diets do have a basis in fact. Some carbohydrates cause you to store fat.

The reason some carbohydrates make you fat is because when they hit your bloodstream they cause insulin to be dumped into your bloodstream. Insulin is a hormone that has one primary job. That job is to regulate your blood sugar. Too much sugar in your blood can lead to vision loss, kidney disease and heart disease. So don't listen to anyone that says insulin is a bad thing. Without insulin, we would be in a lot of trouble.

High insulin levels do cause an increase in body fat stores. When you eat a food that is high on the glycemic index, your blood sugar soars. This results in large amounts of insulin being dumped into your blood stream. Remember that the job of insulin is to regulate your blood sugar. It needs to do something with the excess glucose (sugar). The easiest thing for insulin to do with it is to store it in your body as fat. In fact, insulin is 30 times more efficient at storing the excess glucose as fat than sending it to the muscles where it would be burned for energy. You can't and don't want to stop this insulin response. So what do you do about it? You need to decrease the need for large insulin dumps.

So how do you do this? You simply stay away from the foods that cause the large increases in insulin. That is where the glycemic index comes in. There are a couple of different indexes available. One uses white bread as a standard, with the white bread rated as 100. The other scale uses glucose at the standard, with glucose rated as 100.

The glycemic index was developed in the early 1980's to assist diabetics. Eating foods that are low on the glycemic index would help them avoid dangerous increases in blood sugar. This will also help non-diabetics with body fat reduction. Staying away from the foods high on the index will decrease the amount of insulin and as a result will decrease the amount of stored fat.

For general health and weight loss purposes it is better to consume foods that have a low GI because they tend to keep your blood sugar levels stable and you store less fat. As a runner there are times when you want high GI foods. When you need quick energy or are recovering from a hard workout, high GI foods will give you quick energy and rapidly replenish your depleted glycogen levels.

Eating foods low on the glycemic index will also help increase your energy levels during the day. When you eat a high GI (glycemic index) food, you get an immediate rush of energy because of the high blood sugar levels. The resulting insulin response removes the sugar from your blood, so you now begin to feel fatigued. Eating foods low on the GI will keep you from going through this roller coaster of high and low blood sugar. Your blood sugar levels will remain more stable throughout the day, which will give you a feeling of high energy all day long.

There are times when you will want to eat foods with a high glycemic index. At the end of a long race, such as a marathon, your carbohydrate stores will be very low. Eating a food that has a high glycemic index will rapidly replenish your carbohydrate stores and will bring up your low blood sugar levels. You will also want to ingest a high glycemic index sport drink or food during your race to replenish carbohydrate stores.

The GI of a specific food can vary. Cooking, especially overcooking foods will increase their GI. The GI of bananas will increase as they ripen. The GI of pasta can vary by protein content, size and even shape.

Each individual will also have a slightly different insulin response to each food. Below is a partial list of the GI of some common foods. This list uses glucose as the standard and has a rating of 100

Glycemic Index Of Some Popular Foods						
Breads	Dairy	Fruits	Grains	Legumes	Pasta	Vegetables
White - 96	Ice Cream - 61	Strawberry - 32	Barley - 25	Soybeans - 18	Whole Grain - 37	Tomato - 38
Waffle - 76	Pizza Cheese - 60	Apple - 35	Buckwheat - 54	Kidney Beans - 27	Angel Hair - 45	Yam - 51
Whole Wheat - 75	Low Fat Ice Cream - 50	Pear - 35	Bran - 60	Lentils - 29	Thick Whole Grain - 45	Sweet Potato - 54
Bagel - 72	Skim Mile - 32	Orange - 43	Cornmeal - 68	Split Peas - 32	Gnocchi - 65	Carrot - 71
Rye - 65	Sugar Free Yogurt - 33	Blueberry - 59	Rice - Not Instant - 70	Black Eyed Peas - 42	White Pasta - 65	Pumpkin - 75
Pumpernickel - 49	Regular Yogurt - 14	Watermelon - 72	Instant Rice - 88	Baked Beans - 68	Brown Rice Pasta - 92	Baked Potato - 85

Training and Nutrition

Runners have different nutritional needs when compared to the typical sedentary person. Running burns a lot of calories. Most of those calories are coming from carbohydrates. You are also using some of your protein and fat stores.

Carbohydrate Needs

All athletes have days when they feel sluggish and tired. Their muscles feel weak and performance is impaired. Many times, this is caused by a low level of glycogen, which is the stored form of carbohydrates.

Low glycogen levels can be caused by low intake of dietary carbohydrates, increased levels of training or a combination of the two. As highly active individuals, runners need a higher than normal intake of carbohydrates.

The average diet for sedentary individuals contain around 45% to 50% carbohydrates. This equals about 4 to 5 grams of carbohydrates per kilogram of body weight. For an actively training runner, this level is usually not sufficient to avoid glycogen depletion. When engaged in a moderate intensity training program, a diet consisting of 60% to 65% carbohydrates will help prevent low glycogen levels. Most beginning level runners are training at low to moderate intensity with a least two days off per week. At this level the 60% to 65% carbohydrates along with two rest days per week will allow muscle and liver stores of glycogen to remain a sufficient levels. Approximately 6 to 7 grams of carbohydrates per kilogram of body weight will supply the needed carbs.

As your training quantity or intensity increases, you should increase your carbohydrate intake accordingly. As you add speedwork, interval training, lactate threshold training and long runs, your carbohydrate needs increase greatly. During these periods of intense training, you should eat 8 to 10 grams of carbohydrate per kilogram of body weight. This should amount to approximately 65% to 70% of your total daily calories.

To convert your weight from pounds to kilograms simply divide your weight by 2.2046. For example if you weigh 150 lbs., divide 150/2.2046. This equals 68.03 kilograms. If you are in a heavy training period and want to consume 9 grams of carbohydrates per kilogram of body weight, simple multiply 9 x 68.03 which equals 612 grams of carbs as your target intake.

Now that you know how to do it, I will save you some time. 6 to 10 grams per kilogram of body weight equals 2.7 to 4.5 grams per pound of body weight.

All packaged foods will list the number of carbohydrates per serving. Most fast food restaurants have either a listing in the facility or a web site where you can find the nutritional breakdown of their foods.

Complex or Simple Carbohydrates

All carbohydrates are sugars. Simple sugars are very basic structures, the most common of which are glucose, fructose and galactose. When glucose and fructose are combined they form table sugar. Complex carbohydrates are formed when there are two or more glucose molecules connected together. Complex carbohydrates can become very large with many connecting molecules.

Simple carbohydrates will enter your bloodstream more quickly and can be utilized for energy or stored as fat more quickly and efficiently. That is why sports drinks contain a high level of simple sugars. The carbohydrates are more quickly available for your working muscles go grab on to and use.

While simple carbohydrates are the wise choice when you are in the middle of a long and strenuous activity, such as running a marathon, they are not the best choice for everyday nutrition.

Complex carbohydrates contain many more nutrients than simple carbohydrates. They also are processed more slowly than simple carbohydrates. If you flood your bloodstream with simple carbohydrates when your muscles don't require immediate energy, your body will store the excess energy as fat (after topping off all carbohydrate stores). The complex carbohydrates are processed at a more gradual pace and do not result in a high percentage of storage as fat.

Protein Needs

Athletes need a higher intake of protein than sedentary individuals. Beginning runners especially need a slightly higher protein intake in order to support increases in muscle mass, aerobic enzymes, red blood cells and myoglobin, which carries oxygen in your blood.

Most guidelines recommend taking in 1.2 to 1.4 grams of protein per kilogram of body weight. That equals .55 to .65 grams per pound of body weight. As a percentage of total calories, that equates to roughly 12% to 15% of your total calories.

Strength training has become an important part of a runners training regime. When you are actively involved in a strength training program, your protein need will rise. When strength training your intake should be 1.6 to 1.7 grams per kilogram of body weight or .7 to .8 grams per pound of body weight.

Fat Needs

The average American diet contains about 37% of calories from fat. This is too much. Unlike carbohydrates and protein, athletes do not need more fat than non-athletes. Fat stores on even the leanest runners are more than sufficient to provide fuel for many, hours of exercise. No more than 25% to 30% of calories should come from fat. Fat intake should not be restricted to less than 15% of calories. Fat in the diet is needed to promote healthy skin and hair, protecting the organs from trauma and to help absorb and transport fat soluble vitamins.

Eating Before Exercise

What to eat before exercise or a race really comes down to trial and error. It depends upon what your system will tolerate and what you are accustom to. I cannot eat anything solid less that 3 hours before exercise. Some athletes can eat a full dinner and have no problems. There are however some guidelines that may give you a starting point.

If you have 3 to 4 hours before a race or workout, a meal of 800 to 1200 calories that contain 200 to 300 grams of carbohydrates have been shown to be a good formula for most athletes.

If you have 1 hour or less before your activity, the studies show mixed results. Eating carbohydrates that are high on the glycemic index, an hour or less before exercise, have been shown to result in low blood sugar and a high rate of fatigue. On the flip side, eating a small meal or less than 200 calories, containing carbohydrates that are low on the glycemic index, seem to have a positive effect.

It is even more important to get some nutrition if you are exercising or racing first thing in the morning. The overnight fast can result in low levels of carbohydrates in your body.

Eating During Exercise

During short (less than one hour) races or exercise sessions, you will not need to eat or drink sports drinks. Hydrating with water will be sufficient.

During races longer than one hour, your carbohydrate needs are 30 grams to 60 grams per hour. That equals about 120 to 240 calories per hour. During a race or training run, you need the carbohydrates to act quickly. In this case you need something very high on the glycemic index. The best substance is glucose. That is why most sports drinks contain glucose. It gets into your blood stream quickly and can start providing energy and replenishing depleted carbohydrate stores.

Do not wait until an hour has gone by to start consuming carbohydrates. You should take in the carbs before your start and continue to consume them every 15 minutes. If you wait too long, your carbohydrate stores will be too depleted for you to catch up.

Eating After Exercise

After exercise or a race, you should take in around 1.5 grams of carbohydrates per kilogram of body weight. This equals .7 grams per pound of body weight. Eat or drink the carbs within 30 minutes of the end of the activity. Your muscles will be clamoring for the carbohydrates and will latch onto them quickly and aid in your recovery from the race.

The carbohydrates are the most important nutrients for recovery, but a small amount of protein will also help in muscle repair.

Fluid Needs

Before you start to exercise, drink 12 to 24 oz. of water or sports drink. If your exercise session is going to be less than an hour, water is fine. If it is going to be more than an hour, use the sports drinks. You will need the carbohydrates and electrolytes that the sports drinks contain.

During the race or exercise session, drink 6 to 12 oz. every 15 minutes. Again, if your race is less than an hour, water will work just fine. If it is more than an hour, use the sports drinks. Do not wait until you feel thirsty to drink. When you begin to feel thirsty, you are already dehydrated.

I cannot emphasize enough the importance of consuming sports drinks, which contain sodium, before and during any activity lasting longer than one hour. Hyponatremia is a dangerous condition caused by low levels of sodium in the blood. This is caused by drinking only water, which can dilute the blood. Some marathoners and triathletes have died from this condition after consuming only water during the long race. This problem can be easily avoided by making sure you are drinking a sports drink containing sodium and other minerals when running continuously for long periods of time or in a high heat environment. If you are exercising for less than one hour in moderate temperatures, hydrating with plain water should be sufficient.

Run Safely

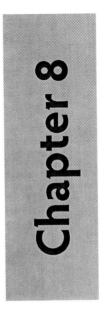

Compared to most sports, running is a relatively safe activity. There is no bike to fall off, you can't drown while you are running on dry land and it is a non-contact sport. But, as with any physical activity, there are some situations that can be hazardous. No worries! With a few precautions you can enjoy your running for many years and avoid most safety problems.

Road Running Safety

The greatest safety concern when running on public roads is the danger of an encounter with automobile traffic. Try to stay off of roads that are heavily traveled. Not only does the traffic present a physical threat, but also the noxious exhaust fumes are health threat. If you must run along heavily traveled roads, try to time your workout so that you avoid the heavy rush hour commutes.

When you are running on roads, try to run against traffic. That way you will always see approaching cars and if a dangerous situation develops you will have a chance to get out of the way. Always run defensively. Look out for approaching motorists because chances are they are not looking out for you.

When you are crossing intersections always advance with caution. Do not assume that the automobile will yield to you. They may not see you or may not care to yield to you. I guarantee that you will lose in a contest with a 2,500 pound piece of steel. Be especially cautious of cars making right hand turns. Many times these drivers are not looking for pedestrians at the intersections. A driver making a right hand turn will look to the left, but rarely to the right. You are usually approaching from the right. If there is a sidewalk or bicycle lane available, use it. Avoid any situation that puts you in close proximity to traffic.

Night Running Safety

You should especially try to avoid running near traffic at night. Stick to side streets with low traffic volume. If you must run in the dark, make sure you wear light colored clothing that will reflect in car headlights. It is also a good idea to wear reflective tape or a reflective vest. Do not wear dark colored clothing. The drivers will be unable to see you at a safe distance. There are also a number of running safety belts, vests and pins that contain blinking lights. That type of product makes if very easy for drivers to see you in the dark.

If you must run at night try to wear or carry some sort of bright light or reflective material. That will make it easier for approaching traffic to see you.

Try not run alone at night. Running with a friend or even better, a group of three or more will discourage any would be attackers. Try to run in well-lighted areas and well-populated areas.

Try not run in parks or urban trails after dark. These areas are usually unlighted. There are few other people that use these trails at night and there may not be anyone nearby to help you if you get in trouble. If you do run at night in secluded areas, carry a good whistle with you. If an undesirable person should approach you, blow the whistle with everything you have. Hopefully, it will scare the assailant away and may attract help.

Do not run in an area that you are unfamiliar with at night. It is easy enough to get lost in a new area during daylight hours. Running at night in an area you are not familiar with is just asking for trouble.

Park and Urban Trail Safety

Running in a park is a generally safe activity. The only significant threats in a well-populated park are other exercisers such as bicyclists and roller bladers. Bicyclists and roller bladers are usually traveling at a high rate of speed and a collision can cause serious injury. Everyone needs to share the park equally, so just watch out for others and enjoy yourself. Do not run in a park at night. They are usually not well lighted nor are there any other people around to help if you get in trouble.

Parks and urban trails can be heavily traveled. You will usually be sharing the trail with bicyclists, roller bladers or horse back riders. Show courtesy to other users for everyone's safety.

Many golf courses have trails running through them that are great running routes. If you use a golf course trail watch out for flying golf balls. Golf balls are small, but they pack quite a wallop if they hit you. Don't run on the golf course fairways when they are in use. Not only is it dangerous, but the golfers pay a lot of money to play on the courses and they would not appreciate being held up by a runner.

Run Safely In Hot Weather

Heat illness is most common during hot weather, but can occur even during mild temperatures. Don't ignore the symptoms of heat illness at any time.

If you are running in an area that enjoys high temperatures, you should take steps to avoid heat related medical conditions. There are a number of serious conditions that can result from running in the heat, including heat exhaustion, heat stroke, dehydration and hyponatremia. These dangerous conditions can rear their ugly head at any time, but are especially hazardous when racing and your effort level is high. Take steps to avoid these heat related illnesses and you will safely enjoy your running throughout the hot summer months.

Stages of Heat Illness		
Stage	Symptoms	Treatment
Dehydration	Thirst, decreased urination, loss of appetite, nausea, fatigue	Drink water or sports drinks, shelter from sun and heat
Heat Cramps	Muscular pains and spasms	Hydrate with sports drinks, rest in a cool, shaded place, massage cramping muscles
Heat Exhaustion	Nausea, dizziness, headache	Hydrate with sports drinks, rest in a cool shaded place, use cool wet towels to cool body, seek medical help
Heat Stroke	Disorientation, vomiting, high body temperature, weak pulse, headache, possible unconsciousness, possible seizures	Get emergency medical help, hydrate with sports drinks, cool body with ice or cold towels

Avoiding Trouble

The best way to treat heat illness is to avoid it completely. Here are some tips that will keep you from suffering from any type of heat illness:

• If high temperatures are expected, try to plan your workout for early in the morning when temperatures are at their lowest.

• When running in hot weather, drink a lot of fluid. Take in at least 6 to 12 oz. of fluid every 15 minutes. If your workout or race is going to last longer than 1 hour, drink a sports drink containing sodium and other electrolytes, instead of water.

• Wear a hat. A hat with a brim will keep much of the sun off of your head and face. Many runners make the mistake of wearing a hat with no ventilation. That type of hat will actually trap the heat next to your head and cause more problems that it prevents. Make sure your hat is ventilated or wear a bandana that will wick moisture away from your head.

• Wear sunscreen. Make sure you use a brand that is sweat proof. Be sure to apply sun block to all exposed areas of your skin. Exposure to the UV rays of the sun can cause premature aging of your skin and has been proven to cause skin cancer.

• Wear loose fitting, light colored clothing. Light colors will reflect some of the heat. There are a number of high-tech fabrics available that will wick the moisture away from your body and aid in cooling.

• Warm up, rest and cool down in the shade. Direct sunlight can cause a rise in body temperature.

• If you are planning a race in hot weather, try to get in at least two weeks of training in similar weather. This will help acclimate your body to the higher temperatures.

Dehydration

Dehydration is the most common heat related problem and is the precursor to more serious heat related illnesses. Many individuals are in a constant state of dehydration because they simply do not drink enough water during the day. Drinking coffee, soft drinks, tea and alcohol can also contribute to dehydration because they are diuretics. Dehydration is not limited to hot weather. You can become dehydrated at anytime of the year, but it is most common during warm weather. You probably will not suffer from all or even most of the warning signs during the early phases of dehydration, but if you notice any symptoms, it is time to take the proper precautions.

The average person needs 8 to 12 - eight ounce cups of water per day. An athlete needs more. An active runner should be drinking at least 80 to 100 ounces of water per day. Runners need to drink fluids all day, not just during their workout or race. Thirst is not a good indicator of hydration levels. If you wait until you are thirsty to drink, you are probably already dehydrated! To ensure proper hydration, drink 2 to 3 cups of fluids up until ½ hour before your race or workout. Drink another 8 to 12 ounces immediately before you start the activity. During your race or workout, drink 6 to 12 ounces of water or sports drink every 15 minutes. If your activity is going to last more than 1 hour, drink a sports drink instead of water.

Warning Signs of Dehydration:

dark yellow urine
decreased urination
loss of appetite
muscle cramps
nausea
dizziness
light-headedness
fatigue
irritability
lack of concentration

It is important to replace lost fluids immediately following your activity. Research has indicated that you should drink at least 20 to 24 ounces of fluid for every pound of body weight that was lost. Most of us won't have a scale available, so as a rule of thumb, drink 16 to 24 ounces for every 30 minutes of your activity. Sports drinks are a better choice than water for after-exercise hydration. The sports drinks contain both carbohydrates and sodium, which will aid in your recovery and in restoring lost electrolytes.

If you ignore the symptoms of dehydration you run the risk of suffering from a much more serious heat illness. There are three primary heat related illnesses. They are, in order of seriousness: heat cramps, heat exhaustion and heat stroke.

Heat Cramps

Heat cramps are caused by dehydration and a loss of minerals. This is not a life threatening illness, but can be very painful. The symptoms are cramping muscles, usually in the calf muscles, but can occur in other muscles. By the time heat cramps occur, you are already dehydrated. You should not continue to run because you will not be able to re hydrate yourself during your run. Drink a lot of sports drinks immediately. Massage the cramping muscles. Try to find some cool water or cool towels to cool your body and move out of the sun to a shaded or air conditioned location.

Cramps are an early warning sign of dehydration and other heat illnesses. While cramps by themselves are not dangerous, they are a way your body warns you that something is amiss. Do not ignore this symptom. If you suffer from cramps takes steps to ward off the more serious heat illnesses.

Heat Exhaustion

nausea
dizziness
extreme fatigue
weakness
weak and rapid pulse
heavy sweating
uncoordinated stride
vomiting

Heat exhaustion is potentially very serious. Left untreated it could lead to heat stroke. As with dehydration, you could have all of these symptoms or only one. Do not take a chance. If you suspect heat exhaustion you must stop running and seek medical attention. Until medical help arrives, lie down in a cool and shaded spot with your feet elevated. Drink a lot of sports fluids. Try to cool your body with cold water or cold towels.

Heat Stroke

Heat stroke is an extremely serious condition and can even be fatal. If the symptoms of heat exhaustion are ignored, heat stroke is very often the next step. This condition involves a breakdown of the system that regulates your body temperature. Symptoms include all of the symptoms of heat exhaustion plus:

• Disorientation

• Lack of consciousness

• Coma

• High body temperature

• Bizarre behavior

• Heavy sweating may be present, but usually heat stroke is accompanied by lack of sweating.

Heat stroke requires immediate medical attention. A runner suffering from heat stroke may be mentally incapacitated or unconscious, so many times, bystanders must assist the ill runner. A person suffering from heat stroke should be moved to a cool, shady spot and cooled with towels soaked in cold water or ice until medical help arrives. If the runner is conscious, large amounts of sports fluids should be consumed. Medical personnel will probably administer fluids intravenously.

Hyponatremia

Hyponatremia is literally water poisoning. Most runners are not aware that they can drink too much water. Not only can you drink too much water, but it can also cause a very serious condition and has even caused some fatalities. The symptoms of hyponatremia include:

- Nausea
- Muscle cramps
- Confusion
- Slurred speech
- Unsteady stride
- Disorientation

Hyponatremia is the opposite of dehydration, but it's symptoms mirror those of dehydration. For prevention the World Health Organization advises using a sports drink that has 20g of glucose, 3.5g of sodium chloride, 2.9g of trisodium citrate and 1.5g of potassium chloride per liter of water. Most popular sports drinks meet these guidelines.

Because these symptoms mimic those of heat exhaustion, many runners make the mistake of increasing water consumption, which makes the condition even worse. To avoid this, drink only sports drinks during events lasting longer that 1 hour.

A low level of sodium in the blood causes hyponatremia. When you sweat you lose approximately 2.25 to 3.4 grams of sodium per liter of sweat. During a race, you will average around 1 liter of sweat loss per hour. If you drink only water during your race, you will dilute your blood even more, which can result in hyponatremia. This condition is usually only a problem in activities lasting more than one hour, but can occur in shorter activities.

Hyponatremia can be a serious condition. If you believe you may be suffering from this illness, seek medical attention. Drinking sports drinks and eating salty foods can treat minor symptoms.

Aspirin, ibuprofen and other anti-inflammatory drugs can contribute to the development of hyponatremia. Because of the popularity of these medications among runners, this condition is becoming more prevalent, especially in the longer distances such as marathons, ultra-marathons and triathlons. To avoid hyponatremia follow these suggestions.

•   Drink sports drinks during events lasting longer than 1 hour.

•   Avoid anti-inflammatory medications.

•   Take in at least 1 gram of sodium per hour.

•   Drink at least 6 to 12 ounces of sports drinks every 15 minutes.

•   Increase your salt intake before your race.

If you are running in an area that enjoys high temperatures, you must take steps to avoid heat related medical conditions. Heat exhaustion and heat stroke are serious conditions that can require hospitalization and in some severe cases, cause death.

Drink a lot of fluids when running in the heat. The average runner will lose between 1.5 and 2 quarts of fluids per hour of running. There is a significant chance of heat injury at all temperatures between 70 to 80 degrees. If the temperature is above 80 degrees, plan to decrease your normal pace to adjust to the stress of the high temperatures. Take in at least 6 to 12 oz. of fluid every 15 minutes. If you are exercising for an hour or more, consume a sports drink containing sodium instead of water.

Heat illnesses can rear their ugly head any time the weather is warm. Always be on the look out for signs of heat injury. Signs include disorientation, headache, dizziness, nausea, decrease in sweat rate, paleness or cold skin. If you experience any of these symptoms - STOP RUNNING. If there is an aid station available, ask for help. If you are running alone, stop running and find some shade. Drink water and pour some water over your head to cool yourself. Get help as soon as possible.

Run Safely in Cold Weather

Hot weather is not the only temperature related hazard for runners. Cold weather can also present problems. When the wind is howling, the snow is flying and the mercury in your thermometer is shivering at the bottom of the scale, you have three choices. You can forget about your run and stay nice and warm in your home, you could run on the treadmill or you could venture out into the cold for your daily workout. Skipping your run should be your last resort. Getting in your daily workout is good for your mind and your body. If you have a treadmill, that would be an excellent choice in cold or stormy weather. If you don't have a treadmill you will have to brave the elements if you are going to run. Don't worry. Unless the weather or conditions are extremely hazardous, you can safely run in most winter conditions. There are some winter weather dangers that you should be aware of and take the proper precautions when running in them.

Hypothermia

We all learned at an early age that our normal body temperature is 98.6 degrees Fahrenheit. Your body has a built in thermostat that make every effort to maintain that body temperature. When your core temperature drops, your body will automatically compensate by diverting blood away from your extremities (exercising arms and legs) and sending it towards your core. That is why extreme cold will adversely affect your running performance.

Hypothermia occurs when your body is unable to maintain its normal core temperature. This condition usually only occurs in very cold temperature, but can happen even in relatively mild (above 40 degrees F) temperatures if you become chilled due to rain, water or sweat. There are three stages of hypothermia as outlined in the following table:

Stages of Hypothermia		
Stage	Core Body Temperature	Symptoms
Mild	95 - 97 degrees F	Cold sensation, goose bumps, mild to severe shivering, numb hands
Moderate	90 - 95 degrees F	Violent shivering, stumbling pace, difficulty speaking
Severe	75 - 90 degrees F	Shivering stops, poor muscle coordination, confusion in the early stages followed by unconsciousness and eventually death on the lower core temperatures.

Hypothermia in runners can happen at any time, but you are most at risk when you stop running. When you are running the energy producing processes are generating heat, which helps keep your core warm. When you stop running you are producing less heat. Compounding the problem is the additional heat loss that is caused by the evaporation of body sweat. So be very careful to either move to a warmer environment or put on some dry, warm clothing as soon as you finish running in cold weather.

Frostbite

A cold weather injury that is closely related to hypothermia is frostbite. As I mentioned above, when your body is struggling to maintain its core temperature, it shunts blood away from your arms and legs and sends it to your body's core to keep it warm. The reduced blood flow to your hands and feet can put them at risk of freezing or frostbite. Frostbite causes a loss of feeling and color. The most commonly affected areas are your fingers, toes, nose, cheeks and chin. There are four levels of frostbite. The first two levels, normal cold response and frost nip are not actual frostbite, but are a precursor or warning sign of impending frostbite.

Levels of Frostbite			
Level	Sensation	Firmness	Color
Early Cold Response	Cold/Painful	Normal	Red
Frost nip	May be numb or may have some sensation	Normal	White
Superficial Frostbite	Numb	Soft	White
Deep Frostbite	Numb	Firm	White

Cold response and frost nip are full reversible and are not serious conditions. Actual frostbite is a serious condition and requires immediate attention.

Wind Chill Effect

As wind passes over your body it carries away some of your body heat. The faster the wind, the more heat it carries away. High wind conditions compound the effects of cold weather. For in depth information concerning wind chill factors including a complete wind chill chart go to: www.nws.noaa.gov/om/windchill.

Keep in mind that as runner, you are generating your own wind chill effect. If you are running at 6 MPH you are generating a wind of 6 MPH. This effect multiplies itself when you are running into a head wind. If you are running at 6 MPH into a 15 MPH wind you are actually suffering the effect of a 21 MPH wind. This can work in your favor in you are running with the wind. Using the same example, if you are running at 6 MPH with a 15 MPH tail wind, your wind factor is only 9 MPH (15 MPH tail wind minus 6 MPH running speed = 9 MPH tail wind)

Air Pollution

Running outdoors in an area of high or even moderate air pollution can be hazardous to your health. This is especially true if you have any type of respiratory condition. Air pollution can come from automobile traffic, industrial exhaust, wood or coal burning or even forest fires.

You should avoid running outdoors during times of high air pollution, especially if you suffer from asthma or any other respiratory problem. Check your local air quality index. If the readings are 100 or higher, outdoor running can be hazardous.

Air Quality Index Ratings		
Air Quality Index Values	Level of Health Concern	Symbolizes by Color
0 - 50	Good	Green
51 - 100	Moderate	Yellow
101 - 150	Unhealthy for sensitive groups	Orange
151 - 200	Unhealthy	Red
201 - 300	Very Unhealthy	Purple
301 - 500	Hazardous	Maroon

If you live in an area that often has poor air quality, try to exercise early in the morning before the pollution levels reach its worst. During periods of high pollution, run indoors on a treadmill or indoor track where ventilation systems will filter out the pollutants.

Carry ID

One of the easiest and most effective ways to decrease personal risk when running is to carry some sort of identification. This is something that most runners do not even think about. Most of us just throw on our running shoes and head out the door. During the vast majority of our training runs, everything runs smoothly and safely. But, things can happen. What if you become ill or are involved in an unfortunate accident during your training run and you have no ID? Responding emergency personnel will not know who you are or who to contact. It is not easy to carry ID. Most running outfits do not have pockets to carry identification.

Where Should You Run?

Chapter 9

One of the great things about running is that it can be done almost anywhere and at almost anytime. All you have to do is lace up your shoes and head out the door. We all have our favorite places to run. Some of us enjoy the solitude and tranquility of a trail run in the forest. Others may prefer the more sensory environment of a crowded city park. More and more runners choose the comfort, safety and convenience of treadmill running. It does not matter what your preference is. There is always an area for you to run. Here is a breakdown of the more common running spots.

Road Running

It does not matter where you live. You always have access to a road or street. Running on the roads is perhaps the most common place to run. You don't need to drive anywhere and you do not need any special equipment. Just put on your shoes, open the door and away you go. While roads and streets are readily available, they do present some challenges that you need to be aware of.

Concrete roads are very hard and unforgiving. If you run on a concrete surface all of the time, your joints are probably going to take a beating. You can minimize the risk by using proper running form. See the chapter on running form an in-depth discussion of form and mechanics.

The road is one of the most convenient places to run. Asphalt roads are softer than concrete and easier on your joints. Always run defensively. Watch out for automobile traffic.

Asphalt road surfaces are a little softer than concrete surfaces and are easier on your joints and muscles. Try to avoid streets that have a severe side slope. The slope will add additional stress to your hips, knees and ankles. It will also increase the chance of turning an ankle.

When running on public roads, you must be very cautions of traffic. Look out for approaching cars, because there is a good chance that they are not looking out for you. Be especially careful of turning cars. They are often looking at other automobile traffic and not looking for pedestrians.

Try to avoid streets with heavy traffic. The traffic presents the obvious physical danger, but the fumes also present a medical danger. If you run at night, choose well lighted roads and wear light colored clothing with reflective materials.

Parks

I believe that running in a park is the most enjoyable place to run. There are many other runners to keep you company. Usually, there is water, shelter and toilet facilities available. Many parks have dirt or cinder trails available to run on, which will be nice and easy on your joints and muscles. Parks are an excellent location for doing longer training runs. You can usually find a good loop run.

With a loop run, you can easily talk yourself into doing one more loop even when you are becoming fatigued.

You should be able to find a park trail to run on just about anywhere. They are numerous urban parks in all cities and towns. Avoid running in parks alone after dark. They are usually not well lighted and there are not a lot of other people around to help if you get in trouble. If your park not close to home you should bring water, food and extra clothing with you. A towel will also come in handy for drying off when you are done running. A large towel will also be useful for keeping your car seats dry and clean.

Urban Trails

Most towns and cities have bike or walking trails that sometimes go for many miles. An urban trail has a lot of appeal because you get to see a lot of different parts of your town or city. These trails may be loops or just long "out and back" trails. If it is an "out and back" trail, be sure to remember that if you run 30 minutes out, you will have a 30 minute run back, so plan accordingly. Be sure to carry water with you on this type of run. There may or may not be water available on the trail. If you live in a large city or town, there is probably an urban trail map available. Check with your area bookstores or chamber of commerce for any available maps.

Urban trails are very popular places to run in cities. These trails are sometimes heavily used by cyclists and roller bladers.

The surface of urban trails can be dirt, cinder, asphalt or concrete. You are sharing these trails with other runners, bicyclists, walkers and possible horseback riders. Run with courtesy. Allow room for other users to pass. Just as with parks, do not run on these trails after dark. They are usually unlighted and seldom used at night. There will probably be no one around to help you in case of trouble.

Cross Country

Runners can go anywhere. You don't need any special facilities or trails. Cross-country running can be exhilarating. You just head out in any direction and run. If you run cross-country make sure you are very familiar with the area you are running in. It is easy to get disoriented without marked trails. Do not run cross-country in a remote area that you are not familiar with. They charge you for costs of search and rescue! Take plenty of water with you since there will be no water stops along the way. You should wear trail running shoes if you are running over rough or uneven ground.

If you are going to run cross country for a long distance, dress appropriately. Dress in layers and carry a jacket. Storms can blow up fairly quickly. You do not want to get caught unprepared in bad weather.

Indoor Tracks

Many gyms and fitness centers have indoor running tracks. Running direction is usually reversed every other day to avoid the risk of injury. Always follow the specified running direction

Many health and fitness facilities have small indoor running tracks. These tracks usually range from 1/20th to 1/10th of a mile. This is a convenient place to run, since you have access to strength training equipment and showers. If you run on these tracks be sure to reverse direction each time you run. The tight and frequent turns of these tracks can cause some hip and knee problems if you run the same direction all of the time.

A track that is banked in the turns can help prevent this problem.

Most facilities direct you to run in a certain direction on different days. Follow the directions as a courtesy to other users. It would be a chaotic situation if runners were all running in different directions.

Outdoor Tracks

Most of today's regulation outdoor tracks are 400 meters or approximately ¼ mile in length. Some of the older tracks may be 440 yards long. These tracks are available at most high schools and colleges. The surface can be dirt, asphalt, concrete, tartan or a rubberized surface. Try to find a tartan or rubber like surface. This type of track is a dream to run on. Outdoor tracks are a great place for doing any type of work out. They are especially good for doing speed work. You

For courtesy and safety reasons it is important to follow proper etiquette when running on an outdoor track

will know exactly how far and how fast you are going. Bring plenty of water with you. You can place it in the infield while you run. Another advantage to outdoor tracks is you are never far from your car or shelter if bad weather or an emergency should arise.

If you are alone on the track, you can run in either direction and at any position that you wish. Usually, there will be other runners on the track. There is a track etiquette that you should follow when sharing with other users. Always run in a counter-clockwise direction. Faster runners will run on the inside lanes and slower runners or walkers in the outside lanes. If the track is busy and you are running in the inside lanes, do not be surprised if you hear someone behind you yell "track!" The runner is telling that they are coming up quickly behind you. If that happens look behind you and move to the right to allow the faster runner to pass safely. Show courtesy to your fellow runners. Following this system will allow everyone to enjoy their workout.

Treadmills

A treadmill is the most valuable type of exercise equipment a runner can own. If the weather is bad or if you are short on time, you can just hop on your treadmill and away you go. Most treadmills can be elevated to simulate hill running and more closely match the intensity of running outside. Many treadmills have a variety of preset programs that will automatically change pace and elevation. If you place your treadmill in front of a television, you can pop in a movie or watch you favorite program while you are running. Putting a fan in front of the treadmill will help keep you cool. Most heath and fitness clubs will have several treadmills for your use. I have written a book available titled "Treadmill Training for Runners". This is an excellent reference for treadmill runners. It includes information on how to run on a treadmill, buying and maintaining a treadmill, treadmill running mistakes and also has many useful treadmill workouts.

Running Form

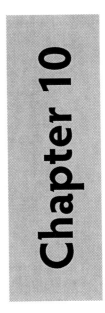

One often overlooked subject when learning to run is your running mechanics or running form. Many beginning runners make the assumption that running form is only important for competitive athletes. That assumption is wrong. It is just as important for a new runner to learn proper running mechanics. In many ways it is even more important for a beginning runner to learn proper form. Learn it now and you will avoid picking up bad running habits that can cause you to become injured, frustrated and an inefficient runner.

Everyone's form looks a bit different. Even among the elite, world class runners, you will see many different specific running styles. Some run low to the ground with little knee lift while others run powerfully, with high knee lift and a strong kick. Some athletes run with a slight forward lean and some run very upright.

Despite the large variety in specific running forms, there are a number of elements that are common to almost all successful running styles. Each of these elements can be practiced and adjusted. Good running form is not something a runner is born with. It is a learned skill. I have been running for more than 35 years and I am still continually making small adjustments to my form. The science and study of running mechanics can get very complicated and involved. As you progress to more advanced levels of running, your running form will become more and more important. For now you only need to learn the basics of proper running technique that will enable you enjoy your running and minimize your chances of becoming injured.

Foot Plant

The most efficient running style is one in which your foot touches down directly under your center of gravity. Avoid reaching out in front of your body. Reaching out causes you to land heavily on your heel which creates a "braking effect" and places excessive impact on your knees and hips.

One of the most important phases of running mechanics is the position of your foot when it lands on the ground. When you foot strikes the ground it will land either; toes first, ball of the foot first, flat footed or heel first. Most beginning runners and many experienced runners make the mistake of reaching out in front of their body and landing heel first. That type of foot plant is inefficient and can be the cause of a long list of injuries. When you land on your heel, your leg is straight and extended in front of your body. The combination of a straight leg and a hard heel landing transfers a lot of impact through your heel and up through your knee to your hip. The excessive stress a heel strike places on your joints can cause pain and injury to your hips, knee, ankle and foot. Many runner are unaware that shin splints (pain of the front of your lower legs) are many times caused by heel striking.

A heel first foot plant also means you are over striding.

You are reaching out in front of your body with each step you take. When you reach out in front of your body, you will land heel first and will be putting on the brakes with each step. It is like trying to drive your car while pressing on both the gas pedal and brake pedal at the same time. You are wasting energy and making your training run harder than it should be. Landing toes first is not an efficient style for distance running. Toe first landings result in a lot of up and down motion and puts a lot of stress on the calf muscles. Toe running is more appropriate for sprinting than for distance running.

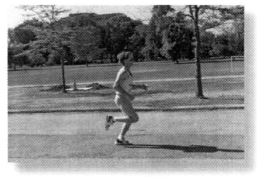

You should always land either flat footed or on the ball of our foot, directly under your center of gravity.

As a beginning distance runner, your most efficient foot plant is one in which your foot lands directly under your hips or your center of gravity. You may land on the ball of your foot or flat footed. The ideal landing position is slightly toward the outside edge of your foot, just behind your little toe. Your foot would then naturally roll slightly inward while pushing off over your big toe. The slight inward roll of your foot is called pronation and provides some cushioning during the running stride. A small amount of pronation is normal and desirable, but excessive pronation can also be the cause of injury and stride inefficiencies. Excessive pronation can be prevented through the use of motion control shoes. That type of shoe has strong heel inserts that stop the inside rolling motion of pronation. While motion control shoes will temporarily solve the problem, it is like putting a band aid on a cut that will never heal. It solves the immediate problem but it not a long term cure. Pronation can be caused by weak muscles in your lower leg or stride inefficiencies. Doing some barefoot walking and running will help strengthen the ankle and foot stabilizing muscles in your lower leg. Doing exercises and drills on an unstable surface such as a wobble board or stabilization pads can also help with this problem. If you pronate severely I would suggest consulting with a physical therapist to find out of there are alternatives to motion control shoes in your specific case.

Posture

Years ago, when I was first learning how to run, I was taught to run with a very upright and straight posture. I was told not to lean forward or backward. Nearly every coach taught that same technique. They coached that way because it was the way they learned to run. I ran successfully using that technique in the early stages of my career but as I advanced to longer, more difficult training runs and higher levels of competition, that technique was no longer adequate. I began suffering from back pain and leg injuries. Running became more difficult and my enjoyment level plummeted. So, I made changes. If you watch world class runners on television, you will notice that they appear to run with no effort. They seem to be gliding smoothly along the road or track. I watched the most successful runners. Nearly all of them run with a straight and erect back, but they lean forward very slightly. This very slight forward lean gives

Efficient running form is all about balance. You want enough forward lean to promote forward momentum but not so much that it will cause a falling, stumbling motion. Some runners find it helpful to visualize their upper body as a jockey riding on a their lower body, which is the horse. Try to keep your body balanced over your legs.

them a completely balanced posture. Balance is the key word. You should always feel as if your upper body is in balance above your hips.

When you are standing still your upper body is very straight and balanced on top of your hips. Go ahead and try this. Stand up and feel your body. Lean your body forward and backward. When you lean forward you begin to lose your balance in that direction. When you lean backward you feel your balance shift to your rear. Only when you are standing with a straight upper body do you feel in balance.

Now start to walk forward. When you being to move shift your upper body very slightly forward. You are leaning into your movement. In a way when you walk you are actually falling forward and catching yourself with your legs. Running is the same. When you run you need to lean forward to keep your body balanced over your hips. If you kept your body straight your balance would be shifted to the rear of your body. You would not be able to continue the action of "falling forward". You would have to reach out in front of your body and pull your legs back to create forward motion. That would make your running more difficult and inefficient.

The most efficient posture is one that is upright and relaxed with a slight forward lean. Your chest should be out and your shoulders back. If you lean too far forward you will begin a stumbling, high impact stride. You will also put excessive stress on your knees and back. A backward lean will cause you to over stride and land heavily on your heel, which will also stress your knees, hips and back. A visualization that may help is to imagine your hips and legs being a motor. You just want to keep your upper body balanced over your motor.

Keep your hips pressed forward and your butt tucked in. Visualize standing face first against a wall. Press your hips forward so that the bones of your hip touches the wall. Running with your hips forward will help your knee lift higher, with less effort.

Another common form error is called "sitting in the

bucket". This is especially common among beginning runners. This style is caused by the hip and butt being pushed back, into a slight sitting position. This causes your feet to be in front of your body with a very weak push off behind your body. Keeping your hips pressed forward will eliminate this form fault.

Keep your body as relaxed as possible. Tense muscles will slow you down and force you to work harder. Concentrate on keeping your shoulders, jaw, torso and legs nice and loose.

Stride Length

The most common form flaw I have observed in runners I have coached is over striding. Forcing a long stride length will not improve speed or running efficiency. Just the opposite happens. Over striding will result in reaching out in front of your body with your foot and landing heavily on your heel. This will cause the braking action that I mentioned earlier. In a proper stride, your foot should land directly under your body with every step. Concentrate on running with a quick and light stride. Your stride should be like a rotary motion with your foot landing directly under your center of gravity at the bottom of each cycle. Over striding is a form flaw, but in order to run as efficiently as possible, you must extend your stride to its maximum, without over striding.

You should increase your stride length by opening up your stride or making "bigger circles" with your feet and legs. Do not reach out with your forward foot, but allow the forward momentum of your body to "catch up" with your forward foot so that no braking action is initiated. Your forward foot should land directly under your body. If you reach out with the forward foot, you will land on your heel and initiate a braking action with each step. This will excessively stress your knees, hips and back, in addition to slowing you down.

Stride Mechanics

All of your effort should directed forward. There should be very little up and down motion. Runners that bounce or hop when they run are wasting energy. They are also putting excessive stress on the knees, hip and back. You should feel as if you are gliding along. Imagine you are running with a beanbag on your head. If you bounce too much the beanbag will fall off.

Your stride should be quick and light. Visualize trying to sneak up on someone while you are running. Your steps should be light and quiet. If your steps are heavy and noisy, you are running with too much up and down motion, or are leaning forward too much.

You should not exaggerate your knee lift when running long distances. A high knee lift is much more important when sprinting or when running hard for the finish line. An exaggerated knee lift will require the use of too much energy to maintain for a long period of time. Knee lift is a very misunderstood term. Many believe that knee lift means to lift your knee straight up, which results in a bouncy, up and down motion which wastes a lot of energy. A proper knee lift should feel like you are driving your knee forward, not up. A forward knee drive will result in a low to the ground and efficient forward running motion.

To initiate your foot plant, slightly pull your lead foot back gently so that it will match the speed of the ground moving under your body. That way you will avoid any braking action and will run very smoothly and efficiently. Immediately after your foot plant concentrate on quickly picking your foot up to continue the cycling motion. It may help to think of your legs moving in a continuous cycling motion, very similar to pedaling a bike. A rather amusing mental cue is sometimes use is imagining I am moving like the cartoon "road runner". I imagine my legs spinning is a continuous circular motion and my body is just going along for the ride.

Arms

The main purpose of an arm swing is to provide balance and coordination with the legs. The arms should hang loose and relaxed, close to the body. Avoid excessive movement. You want to avoid any tenseness in the shoulders. Your wrists should be loose and floppy. Do not clench your fists. Your hands should be held in a relaxed manner. You may try imagining that you are holding a butterfly in your fingers. Do not crush the butterfly. Any tightness in your hands will transfer all the way up your arm.

During the arm swing, your hands should not travel above your chest or behind the midline of your body. Try to avoid crossing your hand in front of your body. Keep your arm swing compact and your elbows at about a 90 degree angle. Do not drive your arms forward. A forward arm drive will encourage over striding. There is only one direction for arm drive - backwards. Driving your elbows back when you run will help you run with a quick, light and efficient stride.

The Twelve Rules of Training

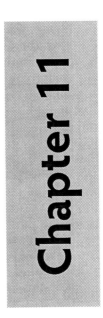

There are as many different training plans as there are coaches. Every successful training program has a number of common rules. I have developed these twelve rules using over many years of coaching experience and hundreds of conversations with fellow coaches. Try to incorporate each of these rules into whatever program you follow and your results will improve.

Begin Slowly

This rule is really like two rules in one. It has two separate, but related meanings. If you are just beginning a training program, start slow and easy. Even if you are in good condition; a new sport or program will stress different muscles and stress joints and connective tissue in different ways. You should let your body strengthen and adapt before you attack it with intense training.

This rule also applies to your daily training runs. If your workout calls for speed work or a moderate intensity run, start out at an easy pace. Your body needs to warm up before you throw any high intensity work at it. If you do not properly warm up, you run the risk of injury. When racing you will usually want to start the race at a pace that is slightly slower than your goal pace. Most athletes perform best when they run "negative splits", which means running the second half of the race faster than the first. If you begin at a pace that is too fast, you may not be able to finish strongly.

Train Your Brain

Your body will attempt to do whatever your mind asks it to do. With any sport or fitness program, there are challenges that you must prepare yourself mentally for. The most strenuous mental and physical difficulties will occur at the beginning of a training program. You should use positive thinking and imagery. Toughen your mind for the challenge that lies ahead and your body will follow to the best of its ability. A major difference between those of us that succeed in a program and those that fail is the ability to overcome the mental blocks and negative thoughts that sabotage our success. Before you can overcome the physical challenges, you must overcome any mental challenges that present themselves.

Train Consistently

One of the most important aspects of training is to train often and year round. It is better to exercise a little all of the time than to exercise a lot infrequently. It is especially important for beginners to train consistently so that the exercise becomes a habit and part of their everyday life. All lifelong runners have made running an important part of their daily routine. Each of those runners have had to force themselves to run everyday when they were first starting. Running or any other form of daily exercise, starts to become more of a daily habit after the first couple of months of the program. The hardest part is the first 30 days. Try to force yourself to do some exercise everyday. Even a walk around the block. Usually, once you get out there and get moving, it becomes easier to keep going. The hard part is getting out the door. If you find it tough to motivate yourself, take heart. It will soon become easier and you will even feel as if you are missing something if you don't get your daily run in.

What happens if you do not train consistently? Fitness gains happen slowly. Loss of fitness happens at a faster rate. If you stop training for a couple of weeks, you will lose the fitness gains of a full month. If you stop running for a couple of months, you will lose almost all of your fitness gains. The popular saying "use it or lose it" is very true when applied to fitness. There will be times when you decrease the amount and intensity of your training as a part of a planned rest and recovery period. During your rest periods, you should still run on a consistent basis in order to maintain a base level of fitness.

Don't Have a Strict Schedule

You should follow a formal training program and have a scheduled routine, but it should not be a strict daily one. A weekly schedule is a better idea. Most training programs will give you a workout for each day. You do not have to follow that schedule day for day. Just try to follow the overall structure of the week. Feel free to move the workouts around to fit your schedule. Try to complete each of the workouts and allow the appropriate rest days, but it is not necessary to strictly follow it each day. With the variables of weather, work and social schedules, health and stress levels, a daily schedule is almost impossible to keep. With a weekly schedule you can fit each work out and rest day in where you can.

There are many times that something unforeseen related to weather, work or social commitments may force you to change or cancel a scheduled workout. If you have a strict daily workout, this may totally disrupt your schedule. With a more informal weekly schedule, you can move workouts around and still meet your training goals for the week.

Set Goals

If you just train aimlessly with no real goal in mind, you will soon lose interest and probably quit exercising. You should set both short and long-term goals. Once you have goals set, your workout will take on new meaning. You will have a reason to go out and exercise.

For beginning runners, possible goals include completing a 5K race, increasing the distance you can run, weight loss, or health and fitness gains. An experienced runner may set goals such as finishing a marathon, improving race performance or using a specific local race as a target. You can use anything you wish as a goal, but you must set one. You will have a much easier time in following a training program when your workouts have a purpose.

Alternate Hard and Easy Days

You shouldn't run at the same intensity every day. If you have a hard workout on one day, either work out easy on the next day or even take the day off. Your muscles and connective tissue will recover and grow stronger on the easy days. If you stress your muscles intensely every day, they will never have a chance recover and grow stronger. Too much high intensity training will also lead to burnout, injury and illness. In the same sense, you should not run always workout at low intensity levels. Adding in some harder running will improve your fitness level more quickly and will keep your program from becoming stale. Most training programs call for higher intensity workouts one to three times per week depending upon your current experience and fitness level.

Train Specifically

Most of your training should be of the type of sport or activity that you are training for. If your goal is to run a marathon, you should tailor your training specifically for the marathon. Since you are a beginning runner, most of your training should be running and strength training. Cross training has become very popular in the past few years. Cross training is simply engaging in other types of training, such as bicycling and swimming. Cross training does have some benefit because it strengthens some muscles that are not used extensively in running. This will help keep your bodies muscles in balance and help avoid injury. But, as a new runner, you will want to concentrate on running. Running should dominate your training. Your most frequent form of cross training should be strength training. When properly done, strength training will take care of any possible muscle imbalances.

When you graduate from the beginning stage and become an intermediate or advanced runner, training specifically become even more important. You will be training for races of various distances from 100 meters to the marathon. The training requirements for each distance are very different. You cannot reach your peak at both the 5K and the marathon at the same time. You must train specifically for each distance.

Use a Periodized Training Schedule

Periodization refers to varying your training during the year. This type of schedule can take on many forms. A high school or cross country athlete has a relatively short racing season. A periodized program for this athlete would be one that concentrates on building a base of easy mileage in its early stages and would gradually increase in speed, strength, specificity and intensity. The athlete in this program would reach a peak or top level of fitness at the beginning of their race season. The training program would then be designed to maintain the fitness level throughout the race season. After the race season there would be a period or rest before starting the sequence again for the next season.

An adult competitive athlete that competes and trains on a year round basis would follow a different periodization schedule. A year round runner will follow a program that include multi-pace running on a weekly basis. They will do a combination of long endurance runs, faster interval training and strength building hill runs during each training week. They will vary their exact program depending upon what they are training for and where they are in their training schedule.

Recreational runners that run for fitness, along with an occasional race, would follow a very different periodized schedule. The scheduled would be less structured, but would still provide for periods of rest, easy runs, strength and speed. The important thing to remember is that you do not want to run at the same intensity all of the time. Too much speed work or high intensity training will lead to burnout or injury. To many easy runs will result in a lower level of fitness and poor race performance.

Listen To Your Body

Your body will always let you know when it needs rest and when it is ready for a hard work out. Do not let an overly strict training schedule force you to exercise intensely when your body is not prepared for it. Weather, illness, time of day, stress level and time of last meal will all affect your bodies ability to perform work. Listen to your body and you will avoid injury and make maximum fitness gains. There will be days when you have a difficult speed workout planned and you just do not feel up to it. You may feel lethargic, tired and sore. This is your body telling you it needs rest. On days like that, just do an easy run or rest completely. You will need to learn your body's signals. As a society, we have made it a habit to ignore what our bodies are telling us. This is a bad habit that running will help you unlearn. However, keep in mind that there are times when you need to push yourself. You will need to learn the difference between a truly fatigued body and lack of motivation. You will always need to push yourself through some motivational struggles.

Cross train

You should obey the law of specificity of training, which was described earlier. However, you should always add strength training to your routine. Strong muscles will help support your joints and strengthen your connective tissue. Almost all running injuries are caused by weak, tight or imbalanced muscles. A properly designed strength training program will strengthen the muscles used in running and improve your overall strength levels. When you start to compete in road races, the strength training will greatly improve your performance.

On your easy or rest days, you can do a different type of exercise such as swimming, biking, walking and skating. This will help develop muscles that are not used in your primary running activity. Be sure that you do not exercise at an intense level on your rest days. The purpose of these rest days are to provide your body with the time it needs to recover and strengthen. If you cross train at too hard of a pace, your muscles will not get that opportunity to recover.

Quality Not Quantity

At one time it was believed that more weekly mileage would result in better performance. Many athletes would run well over 100 miles per week to prepare for relatively short races. Today, we know that it is the quality of your training that matters, not the quantity. You want to train smartly. Excessive mileage or "junk miles" will only result in overtraining, burnout and injury. The mileage required to maximize performance will vary according to the distance you are training for and your current ability level. As a rule of thumb - any miles that you do not have a reason to run are junk miles.

Educate Yourself

Researchers are making new discoveries in the fields of running and fitness every month. Some of these new findings will make previous training methods obsolete and will uncover new ways of training. You should make it a habit to check running publications and web sites on a regular basis for the results of the latest research. You are responsible for educating yourself on all aspects of your physical and mental health.

Train Your Brain

Your brain is a wonderful and powerful organ. It has control over your entire body, including your emotions. Your brain has the ability to convince you to do things that your body is saying you can't. On the flip side, your brain is also able to discourage you from doing things that your body says you can do. Thank goodness you have the final say in nearly all matters. By taking control of your thoughts and attitudes you can take charge of the signals your brain is sending to your body.

An example of your brains ability to override your body's signals involves something called the Golgi tendon organ. This is a sensor in the tendon that attaches your muscle to your bone. The Golgi tendon organ is a protective mechanism to protect your muscles from the damage that could be caused by too much force. If you place so much force or stress on your muscle that it could be damaged, the Golgi tendon organ will encourage your muscle to relax so no damage can occur.

Your mind can override that action. An example would be a heavy steel beam falling on a co-worker at a construction site. Your adrenaline kicks in and you are able to generate a maximum muscle contraction and miraculously lift the beam off your friend. Your mind took charge and over-ruled the natural action of your body. Another example is that of a marathon runner that is able to generate a full speed finishing kick to beat a competitor to the finish line despite being glycogen depleted and having damaged leg muscles.

Running is not only a physical activity, it is also a mental exercise. A positive attitude, the development of mental skills and a well thought out psychological approach to your training is just as important as your physical training. Don't worry, you won't have to make an appointment with your psychologist to develop a mental training plan. As a beginning runner there is just a few key mental skills that you need to master in order to take charge of your running.

Do It For Yourself

I have been coaching for many years and have had clients that met with great success in their running career and others that seemed to struggle. There is always one consistent difference between those that succeed and those that do not. The successful clients run because they really want to. They do it because they enjoy it and want to run for personal reasons. Those that fail want to run because they are being forced to, coerced to or feel like they have to run or exercise. They are not doing it because they truly want to.

There is a wealth of scientific data concerning the behaviors of "want to" versus "have to". Researchers call these behaviors autonomous (I choose to) and controlling (I have to) motivation. These two types of motivation are part of a theory used to explain human motivation called "Self Determination Theory"[1]. According to this theory, autonomous motives come from within yourself and are your own personal choice. In contrast, controlling motives come from, or

1   Ryan RM, Deci El., Self-determination theory and the facilitation of intrinsic motivation, social development and well-being. American Psychologist, 2000,55(1)

you perceive that they come from, external sources and are "forced" upon you rather that being your own choice, using your own free will. To help determine your motivation, ask yourself these questions:

- Why do I want to learn to run?

- Do I want to run in order to meet a personal goal or so I can please others?

- Am I making the choice to run of my own free will or because I am being forced or coerced into doing it?

If you are choosing to run of your own free will and you are doing it because you enjoy it and/or want to do it for the personal satisfaction it gives, you are personally motivated. On the other hand, if you are doing it because you are being forced to do it or feel you must in order to please other people or reach some non-personal goal, you are impersonally motivated.

You will meet with greater success in your running or any other goal you set if you are personally motivated. Personal motivation to learn to run can take many forms, including

- **Improve Your Health and Fitness or Change Your Lifestyle** - This is the most common reason that adults give for beginning a running life. This is a personal motivator in most cases because you are personally reaping the many benefits of running. However, it can also be a non-personal motivator if you are doing it to please someone else or to meet a job requirement. Many of my clients have been members of law enforcement. Many police departments have physical fitness requirements. Some of these clients want to run to meet their departments requirements and keep their jobs. In that case the motivation is impersonal and the clients almost always struggle with the training. They usually will stick with running long enough to meet their short term fitness goals, but because their motivation was not personal, they quit running shortly afterward.

- **Weight Loss** - This reason for running can be both personal and impersonal. If you want to lose weight so that you can have a more healthy, fit body and you want it for yourself, it is personally motivated. On the other hand, if you are trying to lose weight in order to impress or please others, you are impersonally motivated and your chances of long term success will plummet.

- **Interest In or Passion for Running** - This one is the most personal reason for running. If this is your motivator you cannot fail. Getting to this point should be the ultimate goal of every new runner. Even if you are starting to run for another reason, if you strive to get to this level of motivation you will become a life long runner and will enjoy all of running's health and fitness benefits for the rest of your life.

Look inside yourself and analyze why you want to run. Write all the reasons you can think of down on the following worksheet. In the appropriate column note whether it is a personal or impersonal reason and whether the reason is because you want to and choose to or because you feel you have to. You will probably have some of each. If all of your reasons are personal you are in great shape and ready to train. If your reasons are mostly personal with some impersonal you are still ready to train, but work on removing the impersonal reasons from your mind. Only concentrate on the personal ones. If most of your reasons are impersonal you have some work to do. Remember that health and fitness belong to you, not to anyone else. The work you are doing is for you. You are gaining the benefits and putting in the effort. Don't try to please anyone besides yourself.

Reasons for Running Worksheet		
Reason for Running	Do I choose to do this or feel I have to do this	Is this a personal or impersonal reason

The Brain Game

Athletes call it being in the "zone". Everything feels right. Things are moving in slow motion. You see things more clearly. The hoop grows larger when a basketball player is in the zone. Baseball players see the ball more clearly. Runners feel as if they are floating and can run forever. This is the state of mind when your confidence is high, your focus is sharp and your mind is tough. Everything has fallen into place. Your running form is perfect. The "zone" isn't a gift you are born

If you build and maintain a positive self image and eliminate any negative self-talk you can accomplish any reasonable goal and clear any hurdle that you encounter

with; it is learned. You can train your mind for success. Train your mind first and your body will follow.

STIMULUS AND RESPONSE

When performing a sport or challenging exercise, such as running, your mind performs three basic processes. There is an outside event or stimulus which is processed by your brain using your self image which then results in a response. The outside event can be anything from running up a difficult hill or beginning an important race to being passed by a competitor or suffering an injury. Your brain processes this event using your self image. Your self image is basically who you believe yourself to be and how you expect yourself to respond to certain situations. This process stimulates an emotion or response. Any emotion can be stimulated, depending upon your past experiences or self image. The emotion may be positive or negative. Positive emotions will enable you to perform at your highest level and bring about feelings of confidence, challenge, energy, spirit, fun and determination. Negative emotions will disable your ability to perform at the top of your game. Negative emotions bring about feelings of fear, low energy, confusion, depression and lack of confidence. The type of emotion that is stimulated will depend a great deal on your past experiences. If you failed at a certain event in the past and had negative feelings about it, your mind will probably stimulate negative emotions the next time the event arises.

Case Study

Donna H. was running in her first 5K race. She had tried to run in the past and struggled with the training. She ran inconsistently and never really enjoyed it. Donna really wanted to run in this race because her boyfriend was participating and she wanted to impress him by completing the race. Many runners passed her in the first 1/2 mile of the race. She started to feel like she didn't belong in the race. By the end of the first mile she was already fatigued. She started telling herself that she couldn't do this. She was not a runner and she didn't belong there. By the midpoint of the race she had dropped out of the race and swore she would never run again.

In this example the stimulus was the other competitors passing her and the fatigue she felt in the first mile. Her self image was a negative one. She did not feel like a runner and her past experience with running was not a pleasant one. She associated negative emotions and feelings with running. Her response was to expand her negative self talk and drop out of the race.

A few months later, Donna asked me if she would ever be able to run. I told her that she can accomplish anything she would like if she stayed positive and strong. I trained Donna for 8 weeks. In addition to her physical training, we worked on maintaining positive self talk and a positive attitude. At the end of her 8 week training period Donna entered another 5K race. At the start of the race there were still a lot of the faster runners passing her. This time her self talk said "There are runners passing me but that is OK. I have trained hard for this race and I am a runner. It does not matter where I finish. I am doing this for myself". The excitement of the race got the best of Donna and she started the race a bit faster than she should have. She started to become fatigued at mile 2. Donna did not let negativity enter her mind. Instead her self talk said "I am getting tired because I started out too fast. I will slow down to the pace I know I can run and I will finish strong". Donna finished that race and eventually went on to successfully complete several marathons. She became a runner.

STIMULATING POSITIVE EMOTIONS

Successful athletes are able to evoke positive emotions in all situations. In order to bring about a positive response you must block out all negative thoughts and concentrate on the positive. You can do this through self-talk and visualization.

Self Talk

"Imagine" is a powerful word that has no limits. Use your imagination to remove your limitations. When you run imagine your strides as light and quick. Imagine yourself "floating" across the ground. Your body will soon follow the lead of your mind

Self-talk can be either positive or negative. If you are in the middle of an important race and a competitor passes you, negative self talk would be: "I'm failing. That person passed me and is going to beat me. No matter what I do, I can't win. I don't know why I even entered this race." Positive self-talk in the same situation would be; that person just passed me, but he is running too hard. I will stay on his shoulder, let him lead and pass him before the end of the race. I trained hard for this race and I know I can beat him.

For beginning runners, self talk is more related to confidence, past experiences and fear. Common negative self talk for a beginner may be: "I can't run. I am not athletic. I know I cannot do this. I am already out of breath and my legs hurt." A beginner can turn these negative feelings around with this self talk: "This is new to me, but others do it so I know I can. I am going to enjoy my new athletic body. I am breathing hard, but I know this is making me stronger. My legs are feeling the exertion of running and they are getting stronger".

Using positive self talk is a behavior that no one is born with. You must teach yourself positive self-talk. Do not let negative thoughts into your head. Stay positive no matter what happens.

Visualization

Visualization is a mental technique for preparing for an event. It is almost like playing a movie in your head. You are the director of the movie. You should imagine yourself successful completing whatever event you are about to perform. If you are going to run a marathon, imagine yourself gliding effortlessly around the course. See yourself crossing the finish line. If you are about to shoot a free throw, visualize the ball leaving your hand in a perfect soft arc and swishing through the net. This visualization will prepare your mind for positive self-talk and will pre-program your muscles to perform the event. As a beginner, you should visualize yourself as an athlete. Visualize a strong body and heart. Think of having strong lungs and powerful legs. Visualize yourself floating over the pavement with little effort.

Changing Your Self Image

Self talk and visualization will help you to stimulate positive emotions. But, wouldn't it be nice to eliminate the negative emotions? One way to do this is to get rid of any negative self image that you have.

Self image is formed from our past experiences. If you have not been athletically inclined in the past, you may have a negative athletic self image. This is something that you can change. One good way to do this is to make two columns on a sheet of paper. Label one column "current self" and the other column "ideal self". List all of the attributes that you would like to find in your ideal self in the "ideal self" column. Include personal habits, training habits, achievements and accomplishments. In the "current self" column list your current levels in all of the same attributes. Every day, look at that list and practice visualizing yourself with the attributes of your ideal self. Block all of the negative images out and visualize only the habits and attributes of your ideal self. Do this several times per day. You will find that you will eventually become your ideal self and your negative images will disappear.

Self Image Worksheet	
Current Self	Ideal Self

Setting Your Training Pace

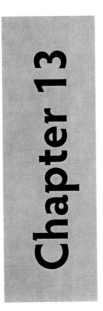

One of the first questions you may have when starting a running program is - How fast should I be running? There are three major methods of determining your training pace - Heart rate training, training by recent race times and training by your rate of perceived exertion. Each has advantages in certain situations. Here are the basics of each type of training and some recommendations.

Heart rate training

Training by heart rate has become very popular over the past several years. When training by heart rate, you wear a belt around you lower chest that has a sensor built into it. The sensor sends heart rate data to a receiver that you wear on your wrist, similar to a watch. You monitor your heart rate by checking the wrist receiver. Heart rate training is based upon two heart rates - your maximum heart rate and your target heart rate.

Your maximum heart rate is the maximum rate at which your heart will beat. This can be determined by a monitored treadmill test or can be estimated with the formula of 220 minus your age. If you are 40 years old, your estimated maximum heart rate would be 220 - 40 = 180 beat per minute.

Your target heart rate is a range of rates that your training program will specify for each workout. You will run at a pace that elicits the desired heart rate. You will either slow down or speed up in order to keep you heart rate at the desired level. The theory is that each of the different types of workouts - easy runs, speed workouts, lactate threshold runs, hill workouts; are best performed at a specific heart rate level.

Target heart rate is calculated using one of several formulas. The two most commonly used are the percentage of maximal heart rate and the Karvonen formula.

Percentage of Maximal Heart Rate

This formula is maximum heart rate x desired training percentage x 1.15. The formula uses a multiplier of 1.15 because studies have shown that a straight percentage of maximal heart rate results in a training heart rate that is too conservative. For example, our 40 year old athlete will have an estimated maximum heart rate of 180 beats per minute. If this athlete wanted to run at a pace that results in a heart rate of 70% of maximum heart rate, the formula would be as follows:

An easy way to monitor your heart rate is through the use of a chest strap monitor and wireless wrist watch style read-out

180 x 70% = 126
126 x 1.15 = 145 beats per minute.

In this example, the target heart rate for your training run would be 145 beats per minute. Your target heart rate will vary according to your fitness level and what type of workout you are doing. It may vary from 50% of your maximum heart rate to 90%.

Karvonen Formula

The Karvonen formula is similar to the percentage of maximal heart rate. The difference is that the Karvonen formula incorporates the resting heart rate. Resting heart rate is the rate that your heart beats when at rest. It is best measured just before getting out of bed. Measure your pulse at your wrist or neck. Count the number of beats in 10 seconds and multiply by 6. This will give you the beats per minute.

The Karvonen formula is a more accurate method of estimating your maximum heart rate because it incorporates your resting heart rate into the equation.

The Karvonen formula is maximum heart rate - resting heart rate x desired intensity + resting heart rate. Using the same 40 year old, desiring an intensity of 70% of maximum heart rate, with a maximum heart rate of 180 bpm and a resting heart rate of 80 beats per minute, the formula would be as follows:

180 - 80 = 100   100 x 70% = 70   70 + 80 = 150 beats per minute

The physiological difference between the two methods is heart rate reserve. The Karvonen formula factors in this reserve which is basically the reserve of the heart to increase its output. Both formulas are very commonly used. Of the two, the Karvonen formula is usually the most accurate.

Advantages and Disadvantages

One of the most common errors committed by beginning runners is running too hard on easy run days. Heart rate training offers the advantage of not letting you run harder than you should be on your easy days. You can set the monitor to alert you if your heart rate goes too high.

The main disadvantage of heart rate training is a lack of accuracy. Estimated maximum heart rates are based on statistics that have a built in variation of up to 19 beats per minute. This means that if you are exercising at 70% of your maximum heart rate, you may be working out at up to 17 beats per minute too fast or too slow. There are many people who can exercise comfortably at up to 36 beats faster than the recommended maximum and those who must keep their heart rate well below the recommended maximum. Your training heart rate will also vary. High heat conditions, dehydration, fatigue, stress, illness and medications can all cause your heart rate to increase, which will decrease the accuracy of heart rate training. Your heart rate will also increase in the last half of workouts or races due to a condition known as cardiac drift.

Training by Current Race Times

Training by current race times is an accurate way to determine training pace. As a beginning runner you can use this method after completing your first race. Until then you should use perceived exertion or heart rate methods.

Determining your pace from current race times is by far the most accurate way to judge training pace. But, there is a rather obvious problem with this system! As a new runner you probably have not competed in any local road races, so you don't have the data to use. Even though you probably can't use this system, I want to make aware of how to use it. Later in your running life you should use this system because it adjusts as you become fitter and faster.

If you complete your 5K races at the maximum intensity that you can maintain, you are running at just over your anaerobic or lactate threshold, which is the pace at which you begin to use more energy than your body can supply aerobically. In a 10K race you are running just under, at, or just over your anaerobic threshold pace. Using your race pace as a guideline, you can calculate a relatively accurate training pace for each type of workout that you do.

If you choose to use the heart rate method to judge your training pace be sure to keep in mind that it is a rough estimate only and that there are a number of factors that can affect the accuracy of this method.

The advantage to this type of training is that it is customized to each individual, instead of relying upon general statistical data. The most useful advantage is that this system adjusts itself to your current level of fitness. As you fitter and faster your training paces increase accordingly. If you take some time off and lose a bit of fitness your training paces will adjust downward to meet your new level.

The disadvantage of race time training is that you must consistently compete in races. You must also compete at a level that is up to your maximum ability in the races. Since you are new to running you have probably not completed enough races at your best intensity, to use this method. You will have to compete in races on a consistent basis in order to get updated feedback on your race times. As your race times improve, you will increase your training pace. If your race times decrease, you will also decrease the pace of your training runs. Keep this method in mind and consider using it once you have completed a few local road races.

Training By Rate of Perceived Exertion

Listening to your body has a lot of advantages. There are more variables involved in how fast you should run than just heart rate. Your stress level, physical health, emotional health, temperature, humidity, the time of day, the last time you ate and what you ate, all contribute to the intensity at which you should run. If you listen to your body, it will tell you all of these things.

The rate of perceived exertion (RPE), also know as the Borg scale, was developed by Swedish physiologist G.A.V. Borg. This scale rates exercise intensity from 5 to 20 depending upon how the athlete feels or perceives his or her effort. The effort ratings range from very little effort to maximal effort. Using the chart may take a little practice but once you are comfortable and familiar with the various paces it can be a fairly accurate way to judge your training pace.

Rating of Perceived Exertion			
Rating	Perception of Effort	Rating	Perception of Effort
5	Very Little	13	Somewhat Hard
6	Minimal	14	Somewhat Hard +
7	Very, Very Light	15	Hard
8	Very, Very Light +	16	Hard +
9	Very Light	17	Very Hard
10	Very Light +	18	Very Hard +
11	Fairly Light	19	Very, Very Hard
12	Comfortable	20	Maximal

The Borg RPE scale, while very useful can be a bit hard to follow with the various ratings of hard, somewhat hard and hard+. To makes things a little easier I have adapted the scale to a more user friendly version.

Beginning Runner's RPE Scale			
Rating	Perception of Effort	Rating	Perception of Effort
5	Lounging in the hammock	13	Running harder to catch up with the dog. You are starting to breath noticeable harder
6	Reaching for a cold drink from the hammock	14	Running away from a small dog chasing you. Breathing hard but still able to talk
7	Sitting up to reach for a cold drink	15	Running from a medium dog chasing you. Breathing even harder but still able talk
8	Walk across the lawn to get a cold drink	16	Big dog chasing you. Breathing heavier. Talking becoming difficult
9	A walk in the park	17	Pack of dogs chasing you. Breathing is very heavy. Talking becoming impossible
10	Taking the dog for a brisk walk in the park	18	Big bear chasing you. Very heavy breathing
11	The dog taking me for a very brisk walk in the park	19	Big bear chasing you uphill. Very heavy breathing
12	Running easy to keep up with the dog	20	Big bear just jumped on your back. You are at maximal effort.

If you choose to judge your pace using a heart rate monitor the table below will give you the approximate heart rate training ranges for each RPE zone.

RPE Heart Rate Equivalent			
Rating	% of MHR	Rating	% of MHR
5	20% - 25%	13	60% - 65%
6	25% - 30%	14	70% - 75%
7	30% - 35%	15	75% - 80%
8	35% - 40%	16	80% - 85%
9	40% - 45%	17	85% - 90%
10	45% - 50%	18	90% - 95%
11	50% - 55%	19	95% - 98%
12	55% - 60%	20	98% - 100%

Your RPE will vary depending up the factors discussed earlier. That is the major benefit of this type of training. If your body is strong and rested, you will feel strong and your pace will feel easier. When your body is in this condition, you are able to train harder and the RPE will support this. If you are feel tired and sluggish, it is because your body needs a break. In this condition, your pace will feel harder.

Suggestions

In the past several years, heart rate training and training in the "Zone" has been the most popular method of training. Many runners, especially beginners, have become preoccupied with their heart rate and will blindly follow it no matter how they are feeling. Heart rate formulas are all based on statistics that have built in variations. Your MHR (maximum heart rate) has a variation of up to plus or minus 19 beats per minute. There is another built in variation of plus or minus 17 beats per minute when you are exercising at 70% of your MHR, which is the "zone" heart rate that has become so popular. That means you could be exercising at up to 30 beats per minute faster or slower than you should be. That is a large potential error.

So what is the best training method? I believe that if you engage in local road races on a consistent basis, race pace training is a good way to go. This will keep your training pace constantly adjusted to the pace that will give you the greatest improvement in fitness levels and race times. In the early stages of your training the rate of perceived exertion is the way to go. This will allow you to customize a training plan with the least amount of calculation or time involved. It will be the most accurate gauge of intensity because it will take into consideration, the current health and strength of your body. The heart rate method is by far the most popular way to judge pace among recreational runners and athletes. Many

In this book I will be using the perceived exertion method for indicating pace. I believe that it is the most accurate method for a beginning runner and it is also the most convenient because it does not require any additional equipment

personal trainers and coaches also rely on the heart rate method, which I believe is a mistake due to the inaccuracy of that method. If the heart rate method is no accurate why is it so popular? There are two reasons - marketing and ease of use. The heart rate method make a lot of money for the fitness industry. There are many companies making heart rate monitoring equipment and hundreds of books showing you the heart rate technique. They don't like the other methods because you don't need to buy their equipment or publications. The heart rate method is also very easy to teach and use. You just strap on the monitor and follow the beeps. You slow down and speed up whenever it tells you to.

There is no question that the heart rate method is easy to use and it will give you a close estimate of your training pace but my suggestion is to save your money and run more intuitively using the RPE method. It will be more accurate, it will adjust to conditions and it teaches how to judge your specific pace rather than being a slave to that "beeping" monitor. Later in your running career when you are consistently competing in races you can graduate to the race pace training which will give you your most accurate training paces.

Learn to Run Program - Your First Steps

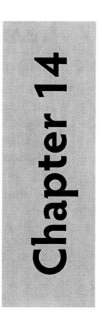

Chapter 14

Now it's time to get the fun started. Keep in mind that running should always be fun. There may be times when you are mentally or physically tired and you don't feel like running. But always remember that running is like play. There is no question that running is a way to improve your health and fitness, but it is also a recreational activity and a sport. Treat it as a fun activity, you will enjoy it more and you will be more motivated to continue. You are doing this because you choose to, not because you are forced to. Every action you take in your life is your choice. Your decision to begin running is a very positive and constructive choice - it will pay you great dividends. You will end up with a fit, toned body and improved physical and mental health. Now - lets get started.

This is an eight week program that I designed for beginning runners. The design of this program assumes that you are a healthy individual with no medical or physical conditions that would limit your participation in an exercise program. You should consult with your doctor before beginning any exercise program.

Learn to Run Program

This program is the starting point for your new running life. This 8-week beginners program is designed for individuals with little or no background in running. The workouts start with only walking and gradually advance to walk/run workouts and finally to all running. If you have already been running or you feel you are a bit more advanced and would like to start with some running right away, choose your appropriate point in the program to start. Just remember not to start out too quickly. It is better to be more conservative at the beginning rather than trying to do too much, too soon.

This beginners program has 6 primary goals:

• **Build strength and "impact resistance"** - When you run the muscles and bones of your legs, hips and feet must absorb the impact of each stride. Your bones, muscles and connective tissues will breakdown slightly and then rebuild to even stronger levels. The gradual increase in running distance in this program will allow your legs to gradually strengthen without causing injuries.

• **Increase your muscular endurance** - Since you are probably new to distance running, your muscles have not adapted to long term use. This learn to run program will increase the endurance of your muscles and allow you to run longer without fatigue.

• **Raise your cardiovascular fitness level** - Your muscles are not the only parts of your body that needs endurance training. Your cardiovascular system, which is your heart, lungs, veins and arteries, also needs to gradually strengthen. Your heart and lungs will build in strength and endurance so that they can provide an adequate supply of oxygen enriched blood to your working muscles.

• **Make you mentally tougher** - Distance running not only requires physical training, it also needs mental training. Your mind needs to toughen along with your body. Running will make you mentally stronger and tougher. This will carry over to all other phases of your life - not just your running life.

• **Exercise consistency** - Running or exercising consistently is one of the most important things you will do. Make running a part of your daily routine and you will improve your physical health, mental outlook and you will maintain a healthy weight. This learn to run program has frequent and consistent workouts for a reason. It is to teach you consistency and help make exercise a part of your life, not just a phase.

• **Build up to 2 miles of running** - Last but certainly not least, a goal of this program is to improve your fitness to a point where you can run over 2 miles without stopping. At that point you are an official distance runner. From there you can train for longer distances or even train to improve your speed and performance. The important thing is to keep running.

The Workouts

Your 8 week learn to run program contains rest days, walking and easy runs. This is a very basic training program and is intended only to increase your fitness level to the point at which you can run 2 miles without stopping. Don't worry about your speed right now. Just concentrate on improving your endurance, increasing your strength and learning to enjoy running. After you complete this initial beginners program, you can move on to more advanced programs that will further improve your speed, fitness and endurance.

You will monitor and adjust the intensity of these workouts using the Rate of Perceived Exertion (RPE) scale. This is a scale that rates your workouts by how you feel. The ratings range from 5 (minimal), such as an easy stroll, to

20 (maximal effort), which is like running as fast as you possibly can.

Easy Runs

Easy runs should be performed at a pace that feels comfortable to fairly comfortable, or a rating of about 12 on the RPE scale. Your breathing should be accelerated but you should never be out of breath at an easy pace. You should be able to carry on a conversation while you are running at an easy pace. If you are breathing so hard that you cannot talk, you are running too fast. If you can sing, you are running too slowly.

Warm up before each workout. Your warm up should consist of about 10 minutes of easy walking. After your workout, gently stretch all of your major muscle groups. Do not stretch until your muscles are warmed up. Stretching a cold muscle can cause injuries.

Rest

Rest is a very important part of any training program. Without proper rest, your muscles and connective tissues will not have an opportunity to recover and strengthen properly. Your daily workouts place stress on your muscles and can even cause very small micro tears in your muscles. Rest days and easy workout days will allow your muscles to rebuild and strengthen. On the days calling for complete rest, do no strenuous activity. On the days calling for rest or cross training, you can rest totally or do some cross training. Cross training can be any activity other than running. You could go for a walk, swim, bicycle or do nothing. It is up to you.

Week One

Your first two weeks of training can involve a lot of emotions. You are probably feeling excited, highly motivated, a bit apprehensive or maybe even slightly scared. It's normal to feel any or all of those emotions whenever you embark on a new venture. Use your positive emotions to fuel your enthusiasm these first two weeks.

Week 1 Beginners Training Schedule		
Day	Workout	Comments
Day 1	Walk for 20 minutes	After this week Day 1 will always be a rest day.
Day 2	Walk for 30 minutes	Walk for about 30 minutes at a comfortable pace. Since this is your first workout, take it nice and easy. Walk at a pace that elevates your heart rate and makes you breath heavier than normal, but you should not be out of breath.
Day 3	Walk for 30 minutes	Same workout as day 2
Day 4	Walk/Run for 33 minutes	Walk for 5 minutes and then run for 30 seconds. Repeat that sequence 6 times. This is your first taste of running. Don't run for more than 30 seconds at one time. Run at a pace that feels fairly comfortable
Day 5	Rest	Take this day as an opportunity to recover from your first taste of running.
Day 6	Walk/Run for 33 minutes	This is the same workout as day 4. Keep your pace fairly comfortable.
Day 7	Walk/Run for 36 minutes	Walk for 5 minutes and jog for 1 minute. Repeat this sequence 6 times. You will make increases like this throughout this program.

Week Two

You got off to a good start in week one. I hope your motivation is strong. If you are struggling mentally this week concentrate on taking that first step out the door. The first step is always the hardest.

Week 2 Beginners Training Schedule		
Day	Workout Completed	Comments
Day 1	Rest	Day Off
Day 2	Walk/Run for 36 minutes	Walk for 5 minutes and then jog for 1 minute. Keep your pace easy. Repeat this sequence 6 times for a total workout of 36 minutes.
Day 3	Walk/Run for 33 minutes	Walk for 5 minutes and then run at an easy pace for 30 seconds. Repeat this sequence 6 times for a total workout of 33 minutes. You are backing off on the run distance today so that your body can recover from your harder workout yesterday.
Day 4	Walk/Run for 36 minutes	Walk for 5 minutes and then jog for 1 minute. Keep your pace easy. Repeat this sequence 6 times for a total workout of 30 minutes. This is the same workout as day 2.
Day 5	Rest or cross train	Today either rest or engage in a non-running activity. Good cross training activities include swimming, bicycling, hiking, tennis, etc.
Day 6	Walk/Run for 35 minutes	Walk for 5 minutes then run at an easy pace for 2 minutes. Repeat this sequence 5 times for a total workout of 35 minutes.
Day 7	Walk/Run for 35 minutes	Walk for 5 minutes and then run at an easy pace for 2 minutes. Repeat this sequence 5 times for a total of 35 minutes. This is the same workout as day 6.

Week Three

This week you are going to continue to extend the distance of the running portions of your workouts. At the end of this week you will be walking 5 minutes and running 4 minutes. Concentrate on staying mentally strong. The excitement of starting a new adventure carried you through the first 2 weeks. Now you need to focus on staying mentally strong and motivated.

Week 3 Beginners Training Schedule		
Day	Workout	Comments
Day 1	Rest	Rest
Day 2	Walk/Run for 32 minutes	Walk for 5 minutes and then run at an easy pace for 3 minutes. Repeat this 4 times for a total of 32 minutes
Day 3	Walk/Run for 35 minutes	Walk for 5 minutes and then run at an easy pace for 2 minutes. Repeat this 5 times for a total workout of 35 minutes. You back off on the distance of your run today for recovery.
Day 4	Walk/Run for 32 minutes	Walk for 5 minutes and then run at an easy pace for 3 minutes. Repeat this 4 times for a total of 32 minutes. This is the same workout as day 2.
Day 5	Rest or cross train	Rest or cross train today. It is your choice.
Day 6	Walk/Run for 36 minutes	Walk for 5 minutes and then run at an easy pace for 4 minutes. Repeat this 4 times for a total of 36 minutes.
Day 7	Walk/Run for 36 minutes	Walk for 5 minutes and then run at an easy pace for 4 minutes. Repeat this 4 times for a total of 36 minutes.

Week Four

You are going to make a big step this week. The running portions of your workouts will become longer than your walking portions. You will also begin to decrease the walking intervals . Your doing great! Keep going and stay strong.

Day	Workout	Comments
Week 4 Beginners Training Schedule		
Day	Workout	Comments
Day 1	Rest	Rest
Day 2	Walk for 30 minutes	You have made a lot of progress in the last week and have placed a good deal of stress on your body. You are eliminating the running portion today for recovery.
Day 3	Walk/Run for 30 minutes	Walk for 5 minutes and then run at an easy pace for 5 minutes. Repeat this 3 times for a total workout of 30 minutes. Keep your pace easy.
Day 4	Walk/Run for 36 minutes	Walk for 5 minutes and then run for 4 minutes. Repeat this 4 times for a total of 36 minutes. You are decreasing your running interval today for some recovery.
Day 5	Rest or cross train	Rest or cross train
Day 6	Walk/Run for 36 minutes	Walk for 4 minutes and then run at an easy pace for 5 minutes. Repeat this 4 times for a total workout of 36 minutes. Today, you will begin decreasing your walking intervals instead of increasing your running intervals. Keep your pace easy.
Day 7	Walk/Run for 36 minutes	Walk for 4 minutes and then run at an easy pace for 5 minutes. Repeat this 4 times for a total workout of 36 minutes. This is the same workout as day 6.

Week Five

Congratulations! You have completed your first month of training and you are doing great. For many beginning runners, the first 4 weeks are the toughest. You have been using muscles that may not have seen a lot of action lately. Now you are feeling stronger both physically and mentally. Stay focused to avoid a let down.

Week 5 Beginners Training Schedule		
Day	Workout	Comments
Day 1	Rest	Rest
Day 2	Walk/Run for 32 minutes	Walk for 3 minutes and then run at an easy pace for 5 minutes. Repeat this 4 times for a total workout of 32 minutes. You are making another decrease in your walking interval today.
Day 3	Walk/Run for 36 minutes	Walk for 4 minutes and then run at an easy pace for 5 minutes. Repeat this 4 times for a total workout of 36 minutes.
Day 4	Walk/Run for 32 minutes	Walk for 3 minutes and then run at an easy pace for 5 minutes. Repeat this 4 times for a total workout of 32 minutes. This is the same workout as day 2.
Day 5	Rest or cross train	Rest or cross train. If you are feeling fatigued use this day for total rest.
Day 6	Walk/Run for 35 minutes.	Walk for 2 minutes and then run at an easy pace for 5 minutes. Repeat this 5 times for a total workout of 35 minutes.
Day 7	Walk/Run for 35 minutes.	Walk for 2 minutes and then run at an easy pace for 5 minutes. Repeat this 5 times for a total workout of 35 minutes. This is the same workout as day 6.

Week Six

You are going to take another significant step this week. The walking portions of your workouts are going to dip below 1 minute. During the last two workouts this week your walking intervals will only be 30 seconds. You are getting very close to completing your initial goal. Don't fall behind schedule at this point.

Week 6 Beginners Training Schedule		
Day	Workout	Comments
Day 1	Rest	Rest
Day 2	Walk/Run for 30 minutes	Walk for 1 minute and then run at an easy pace for 5 minutes. Repeat this 5 times for a total workout of 30 minutes.
Day 3	Walk/Run for 35 minutes	Walk for 2 minutes and then run at an easy pace for 5 minutes. Repeat this 5 times for a total workout of 35 minutes.
Day 4	Walk/Run for 36 minutes	Walk for 1 minute and then run at an easy pace for 5 minutes. Repeat this 6 times for a total of 36 minutes.
Day 5	Rest or cross train	Always rest on this day if you are feeling fatigued.
Day 6	Walk/Run for 33 minutes	Walk for 30 seconds and then run at an easy pace for 5 minutes. Repeat this 6 times for a total workout of 33 minutes.
Day 7	Walk/Run for 33 minutes.	Walk for 30 seconds and then run at an easy pace for 5 minutes. Repeat this 6 times for a total workout of 33 minutes. This is the same workout as day 6.

Week Seven

	Week 7 Beginners Training Schedule	
Day	Workout	Comments
Day 1	Rest	Rest
Day 2	2 x 1 mile repeats or 2 x 1600 meter repeats	Today you are going to try something new. Go to a school track or a trail in your area that you have measured. Warm up with vigorous walking for 10 minutes. Then run 2 x 1 mile or 1600 meter repeats. To do this, run 1 mile or 1600 meters at an easy pace. Then walk 5 minutes before running another mile or 1600 meters at an easy pace.
Day 3	Walk/Run for 33 minutes	Walk for 30 seconds and then run at an easy pace for 5 minutes. Repeat this 6 times for a total of 33 minutes.
Day 4	Run 1.25 miles or 2 kilometers	You are going to try another new workout today. Walk for 10 minutes to warm up. Then run for 1.25 miles or 2 kilometers without stopping or walking. You can do this run nearly anywhere - through your neighborhood, in a park, on a school track or on a treadmill.
Day 5	Rest or cross train	Rest or cross train
Day 6	2 x 1 mile repeats or 2 x 1600 meter repeats	Warm up with 10 minutes of walking. Then run 2 x 1 mile or 1600 meter repeats. Cool down with 10 minutes of walking. This is the same workout as day 2.
Day 7	Run 1.5 miles or 2.4 kilometers	Walk for 10 minutes to warm up. Then run 1.5 miles or 2.4 kilometers without stopping or walking. Cool down with 10 minutes of walking.

Week Eight

You're in the home stretch! At the end of this week you will be running over two miles without stopping! You are now a runner! This should be an exciting week for you. I don't think you will have any problems with motivation and you should now be very strong physically. Don't stop here. This is just the first step in your running life. Set new goals and take on new challenges. Never stop running!

Week 8 Beginners Training Schedule		
Day	Workout	Comments
Day 1	Rest	Rest
Day 2	2 x 1 mile repeats or 2 x 1600 meter repeats	Walk for 10 minutes to warm up. Then run 2 x 1 mile or 1600 meter repeats. Cool down with 10 minutes of walking.
Day 3	Walk/Run for 33 minutes	Walk for 30 seconds. Then run at an easy pace for 5 minutes. Repeat this 6 times for a total of 33 minutes.
Day 4	Run 1.75 miles or 2.8 kilometers	Walk for 10 minutes to warm up. Then run 1.75 miles or 2.8 kilometers without stopping or walking. Cool down with 10 minutes of walking.
Day 5	Rest or cross train	Rest or cross train
Day 6	Run 2 miles or 3.2 kilometers	Warm up with 10 minutes of walking. Then run 2 miles or 3.2 kilometers without stopping or walking. Cool down with 10 minutes of walking.
Day 7	Run 2.25 miles or 3.6 kilometers	Walk for 10 minutes to warm up. Then run 2.25 miles or 3.6 kilometers without stopping or walking. Cool down with 10 minutes of walking

Moving On

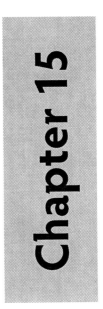
Now that you have graduated from the beginning runner program you may be asking - "What now"? Where do you go from here? That is a very good and important question. How you answer that question can have a great effect on your running future. The most critical thing to keep in mind in answering that question is that you must always have a goal in mind. Don't fall into the trap of just wandering aimlessly without direction. Beginning runners who do not continue to set goals often quit running and lose the fitness that they worked so hard to gain. Don't let that happen to you.

Your next goal can be nearly anything from continuing to improve your fitness to running a 5K race, a 10K or even completing a marathon. No one can tell you what is best for you. Only you can decide what your next step will be. To help you make your decision use the following table which outlines the basic requirement to meet each goal.

Moving On - Future Running Goals			
Goal	Time Requirements	Effort Requirements	Benefits/Risks
Recreational Running/Fun	Minimal - 3 to 5 days per week. 20+ minutes per day	Minimal - mostly easy running	Improved health, reduced stress. Low injury and health risk
Fitness/Weight Management	Minimal to moderate - 4 to 7 days per week. 20+ minutes per day	Minimal to moderate - mostly easy running. Some more intense running and strength training	Improved health, reduced stress, ideal weight, stronger muscles. Low injury and health risk
Run a 5K	Moderate - 4 to 7 days per week. 30+ minutes per day	Moderate - A combination of easy running and higher intensity running/strength training	Improved fitness, improved running performance, stronger muscles. Low to moderate injury and health risk
Run a 10K	Moderate - 4 to 7 days per week. 30 to 60+ minutes per day	Moderate - A combination of easy running and higher intensity running/strength training	Improved fitness, improved running performance, stronger muscles. Low to moderate injury and health risk
Run a 1/2 Marathon	Moderate to high - 4 to 7 days per week. 30 to 120+ minutes per day	Moderate to high - A combination of easy running, long runs and higher intensity running/strength training	Improved fitness, higher endurance, improved running performance, stronger muscles. Low to moderate injury and health risk

Moving On - Future Running Goals			
Goal	Time Require-ments	Effort Require-ments	Benefits/Risks
Run a Marathon	High - 5 to 7 days per week. 30 to 180+ minutes per day	High - A com-bination of easy running, long runs and higher intensity running/ strength training	Improved fitness, higher endur-ance, improved running perfor-mance, stronger muscles. Moder-ate injury and health risk
Become a year round competi-tive athlete	High - 5 to 7 days per week. 30 to 180+ minutes per day year round	High - A com-bination of easy running, long runs and higher intensity running/ strength training	Improved fitness, higher endur-ance, improved running perfor-mance, stronger muscles. Moder-ate injury and health risk

The above table not only gives you some possible future goals but also shows the most logical, efficient and safe progression of your running life. After graduating from the beginners program you can do one of three things.

- Stop running
- Continue to run for fitness or recreation
- Train to compete in running events and races

The first option is not a true option in my mind. You have taken the positive and life changing step of learning to run - now keep going. Running will improve your health, raise your fitness level, increase your strength, decrease your stress, lengthen your lifespan and improve your social life. There is no reason not to continue setting new running goals, so don't even consider that option.

Many runners are not interested in taking part in run-ning events and that is perfectly OK. The physical and mental benefits of running are the reason nearly all run-ners continue to take part in this great sport. Participating in races is just the icing on the cake. So, the next logical step for many new runners is to continue to run on a consistent life long basis for fitness and fun. And always keep in mind that running should be fun. No one is forcing you to do this. You have made the choice to run and it was an excellent choice. Always enjoy your running and rejoice in your God given ability to run.

Recreational Running

This is a broad category. Nearly every runner, no matter what their level or goal is also a recreational runner. Even world class competitive runners also run for fun and recreation. Many new runners move into this category after graduating from the beginners program. The time requirements are minimal and the benefits are high. There is not a lot of structure to a recreational running program. You simply run when and where you would like to. You choose your speed and distance. The goal is to enjoy yourself and maintain your fitness level. The only requirement is consistency. You are on your way to becoming a life long runner so you really should make running a part of your everyday routine. You don't need to run everyday. You certainly can, but to don't have to. There are no requirements. That being said, I think it is very important to run on a consistent basis. I would suggest never taking off more than two consecutive days unless you are injured or ill.

As I mentioned, there is no real structure to a recreational runners training program. But it sometimes helps to have a basic format to follow. Here is a basic one week training schedule that you can follow or use to design your own recreational running program.

7 Day Recreational Runners Schedule

Day	Workout	Comments
Day 1	Rest	A good day for rest is after a long run. Your muscles probably will need it.
Day 2	Easy Run	Run between 2 and 3 miles at a comfortable pace
Day 3	Higher Intensity Run	Run either slightly faster than your easy pace or at your easy pace over hilly terrain. Higher intensity running will improve your fitness even more.
Day 4	Rest	Another good day for rest is after a harder run.
Day 5	Easy Run	2 to 3 miles at comfortable pace
Day 6	Easy Run	2 to 3 miles at comfortable pace
Day 7	Long Run	Start with your longest run in the past 2 weeks. Each time you do your long run add a bit more mileage. This will improve your endurance and fitness. Don't add a lot of mileage at one time. A good rule of thumb is no more than a 10% increase. Increase your long run up to the level that most closely meets your specific goals.

This is only a sample recreational runners schedule. You can design any routine you desire but there are some specifics that your training program should include:

• **Consistent running** - no more than 2 consecutive days off.
• **Hard/Easy sequence** - You should always have either a rest day or an easy running day after a long run or a hard run.
• **Include some higher intensity running** - Faster paced running or hill running will do wonders for your fitness level as well as adding in some much needed variety.
• **Include a weekly or biweekly long run** - You should always challenge yourself with longer distances. Your endurance level will skyrocket and your fitness will follow suit.

Running For Weight Loss

Weight loss is one of the top reasons beginning runners give for starting a running program. It takes a combination of cardiovascular exercise and strength training to maximize your ability to burn calories and maintain or decrease your weight. The cardiovascular exercise, such as running, will burn calories and will also make changes in your body that make you a more efficient fat burner. Muscle mass is where most of the energy is burned in your body. That is why strength training is important. The strength exercises build more of the energy burning muscles. Here is a weight loss training program that I have designed that will burn calories, build strength, improve your fitness and most importantly help you lose or maintain your weight.

This program uses a 14 day schedule. This does not mean that you exercise for 14 days and then quit. You simply keep following the 14 day cycle of workouts for the duration of your program. This program uses three special workouts which I call – The Big Easy, The Fat Buster and The Strength Circuit.

The Big Easy

This workout is simple to perform. Simply warm up and then run at your easy endurance or comfortable pace. You can judge your easy pace using this simple rule of thumb. You should be able to speak clearly but not sing. If you cannot speak clearly you are walking or running too fast. If you can sing clearly you are not moving fast enough

The Strength Circuit

Strength training is an important part of any weight maintenance program. Muscles are the engines of your body. When you build more muscle you are basically making a bigger, more powerful engine. That bigger engine requires more fuel in the form of calories to keep running. So, the more muscle you have, the more calories you burn on a daily basis. This workout combines the benefits of an easy endurance run with some general strength training exercises that will begin to build more muscle and burn more calories. This workout is considered an endurance workout because of the low intensity of the running portions, but it is not an easy workout. You will move between the running portions and the strength portions with no rest. After a warm up, perform this routine, alternating between easy running and a strength training exercise.

- Run or walk for ½ mile
- Push ups for 30 seconds
- Run or walk for ½ mile
- One leg squats for 30 seconds
- Run or walk for ½ mile
- Triceps press ups for 30 seconds
- Run easy for ½ mile
- Core stabilization for 30 seconds
- Run easy for ½ mile
- Bench step ups for 30 seconds
- Run easy for ½ mile
- Biceps curls for 30 seconds
- Cool down for 5 minutes

See the chapter on strength training for descriptions of these strength exercises.

The Fat Buster

Weight loss is a function of calories in versus calories out. If you burn more calories than you take in, on a daily basis, you will lose weight. I am sure that you have read at various times, that if you want to lose weight, you should exercise in the "weight loss zone". No, that is not a black and white horror series narrated by Rod Serling. The "Zone" is an exercise heart rate range of approximately 65% to 75% that is touted by some to be the ideal exercise intensity for weight loss. They tell you that if you exercise at a higher intensity, you are not burning fat. They are partially right, but mostly wrong.

Slow to moderate running is not always the most efficient way to burn calories and lose weight. Higher intensity running will build more muscle, make greater increases in your fitness level, make you a more efficient calorie burner and burn more calories per minute of exercise.

When you are exercising at a low intensity, you are exercising aerobically, which means "with oxygen". When you are exercising aerobically, you are burning both fat and carbohydrates to produce energy. In contrast, when you are exercising as hard as you can, such as when you are sprinting, your body cannot use oxygen fast enough to provide enough energy. At this point you are exercising anaerobically, which means "without oxygen." When you are exercising anaerobically you are burning mostly carbohydrates to produce the energy. The proponents of the "Zone" system do not want you to stray above the fat burning zone because they feel that the goal is to burn as much fat as possible during your workout. That sounds good in theory, but in practice it is the wrong approach. You actually burn very little fat in any one workout. For weight loss, your goal should be to maximize your calorie burn in every workout. To do this you need to include some intense exercise in your run. Why? - Because higher intensity exercise does two important things for you:

• It burns more calories per minute than low intensity exercise.
• It improves your level of fitness and makes improvements in your body at the cellular level that trains you to improve the pace of your easy runs so that you begin to

burn even more calories in all of your workouts. It improves your body's ability to burn fat as fuel.

This workout is designed to increase the calories burned during your run, while maintaining the overall easy qualities of the workout. In this workout you will run for 30 minutes alternating between 5 minutes at an easy pace and short 1 minute repeats at a progressively faster pace.

Fat Buster Workout

- Run at a comfortable pace for 5 minutes.
- Increase your speed to a somewhat hard pace and run for 1 minute.
- Decrease your speed back to an easy pace and run for 5 minutes.
- Increase your speed to a somewhat hard pace run for 1 minute,
- Return to an easy pace for 5 minutes.
- Increase your speed to a hard pace and run for 1 minute.
- Now return to an easy pace for another 5 minutes.
- Increase your speed to a hard pace and run for 1 minute.
- Return to an easy pace for 5 minutes then
- Increase your speed to a very hard pace and run for 1 minute.
- Cool down with a few minutes of easy running.
-

Those three workouts will help you lose weight and body fat. Never forget that one of the most important rules of this or any other training program is consistency. Keep at it. If you combine this weight loss program with a diet composed of reasonable portions of high quality foods you will achieve whatever weight loss goals you have set for yourself.

Running For Weight Loss Schedule		
Day	Workout	Comments
Day 1	The Big Easy	Run 2 miles
Day 2	The Strength Circuit	Perform 1 circuit
Day 3	Rest	Rest Day
Day 4	The Big Easy	Run 2. 5 miles
Day 5	The Fat Buster	1 full workout
Day 6	The Big Easy	Run 3 miles
Day 7	The Strength Circuit	Perform 1 circuit
Day 8	The Big Easy	3 miles
Day 9	Rest	Rest Day
Day 10	The Fat Buster	1 full workout
Day 11	The Big Easy	Run 4 miles
Day 12	The Strength Circuit	1 circuit
Day 13	The Big Easy	Run 3 miles
Day 14	The Fat Buster	1 full workout

Continue this cycle for the duration of your program. As you become fitter, increase the distance of your easy runs. Do not make any sudden increases in mileage. If you increase your mileage too fast, you will risk injury. A good rule of thumb is to make no increases over 10%. The higher intensity running you are doing with The Fat Buster workout, will improve your running speed. As your fitness level increases your running will begin to feel easier at all paces. So, you should always be adjusting your pace. You should be able to perform your easy runs at faster speeds, while maintaining the comfortable pace. The faster speed will equal more calories burned during your easy runs. Also adjust the speed of your higher intensity runs as your fitness level increases.

Training For Races

Some beginner running graduates started to run with the intention of competing in a road or trail race. Some fitness runners also become interested in racing and make that their new goal. Racing becomes the next logical step in your progression. You have gained fitness and strength during your beginners program. Some of you have improved on that through a period of recreational or fitness running. Now you are ready to start racing. Where do your start? What distance should you start with? My suggestion would be to progress from your first 5K to a 10K, a half marathon and finally a full marathon. But, many of today's new runners want to take on the challenge of a marathon right away. That is an admirable goal and one that you can achieve. But before you decide to take on the marathon, ask yourself some questions.

Are You Mentally Prepared For Marathon Training?

I would like to make one thing very clear. Nearly anyone can train for and complete a marathon. I have seen runners of all ages and abilities finish the race. I have seen athletes overcome physical handicaps off all kinds to cross the finish line. There is one thing that all of these athlete's have in common. They are highly motivated and dedicated to completing their goal.

One of my favorite movie quotes is from "The Karate Kid". In that film Pat Morita's character - Mr. Miyagi - asks Daniel, played by Ralph Macchio, if he is ready to learn karate. Daniel replies, "I guess so". Mr. Miyagi looks at Daniel and after a heavy sigh, says: "Daniel-san, must talk. Man walk down road. Walk left side, safe. Walk right side, safe. Walk down middle, sooner or later, get squished, just like a grape. Same here. You karate do "yes," or karate do "no", safe. You karate do "guess so," just like grape."

Marathon training is very similar to Mr. Miyagi's explanation to Daniel about karate training. If you are going to run a marathon, you must be 100 percent dedicated to completing the required training. If you attempt to run the marathon without the proper training, your race will not be an enjoyable experience for you. If you are not fully dedicated to completing your goal or if you are not mentally prepared for the training required, you are setting yourself up for failure.

Before you set a goal of completing a marathon, search inside yourself and be sure that you have the desire, dedication and support that is necessary to complete the required training.

Are You Physically Ready to Train For a Marathon?

I have read many books and training programs that tell you how easy it is to train for a marathon in just a few months. This is true for a runner that has several years of experience and is already at a high level of fitness. But, for new runners, attempting to run a marathon with just 3 or 4 months of training can be physically very difficult, mentally draining and in some cases medically hazardous.

Those accelerated training programs take you from zero miles to 26.2 miles in just a few months. The major problem with that is the fact that a new runner has not built up the base of strength and endurance that is required for strenuous marathon training. You would not teach yourself to fly by jumping off the roof of your house. In the same sense, it is not a good idea to take yourself from zero to 26 miles in a short period of time.

The average marathon runners takes around 42,000 steps during a race. The muscles, tendons, ligaments and joints of a new runner are just not properly prepared or strengthened for that much work. When an inexperienced runner attempts a marathon without a sufficient amount of base training, the results can and often do include: failure to finish, injuries, mental burnout, illness or failure to complete the training. Even many of those that finish never run another marathon because the first one was not enjoyable to them.

A safer and more sensible approach for a new runner would be to first train for a 5K race. After successfully completing the 5K and getting comfortable with that distance, graduate to 10K training and complete a 10K race. At that point the runner has built up a good base of fitness and has gained some strength in their leg muscles and connective tissues. They have also learned whether or not they enjoy this wonderful sport of running. They can now begin a marathon training program and be more assured of enjoying the process and successfully reaching their goal.

This does not mean that a beginning runner cannot train for a marathon. But, in my opinion, 3 or 4 months is not a sufficient amount of time. If you are new to running, try to allow yourself 6 to 7 months to prepare for your marathon. That amount of time will allow you to gradually and safely improve your muscle strength and endurance so that you can reach your goal with a minimal risk of injury.

Whether you decide to run a marathon, a 10K or another 5K, it is important to set a goal and work towards it. You do not need to use a race as a running goal. You could also train for general fitness, increase your endurance, improve your strength, lose weight or get faster. The important thing is to set a goal. Goals are great motivational tools. They keep you focused and on target.

Other ways to stay motivated include joining a running club, getting friends and family involved, running for charity or becoming some ones mentor. Many beginning runners end up getting a fitness or coaching certification and make a new career out of running.

Keep setting goals and always challenge yourself. You will run for a lifetime and reap the benefits of being a lifelong runner.

Become a Competitive Athlete

I have been coaching runners for many years. Some run for the previously touched upon reasons of fitness, weight loss and recreation. There are also many runners that have the long term goal of becoming a life long competitive athlete. This is an admirable and rewarding goal, but it is not for everyone. Your first question may be - what exactly is a competitive athlete? Some have the mistaken belief that a competitive athlete is one who is always in the running for top finishing positions. That is far from the truth. Your finishing position in races has little to do with it. A competitive athlete is a runner who consistently trains to be the very best they can possibly be. They train year round using a varied and specific workout schedule that includes many different types of workouts. Their goal is to always be running at their peak ability.

The time requirements, dedication and effort involved are high, but the rewards are great. The training involved gives a competitive athlete a strong finely tuned body and a mental toughness that can only be obtained through consistent long term training.

If this is your long term goal I would encourage you to start with consistent running and progress through the race distances. Once you are able to run 5K and 10K races without difficulty you are ready to move onto more advanced training programs that include a wider variety of workouts to improve your speed, endurance, strength and power.

Your First Race

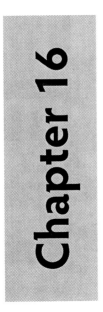

I have taught many hundreds of people how to run during my coaching career. They have been young, old, male and female. Most of them went on to compete in local and in some cases national races. At first, many of my clients had no interest in racing. I always suggest taking up the sport of racing, but many times I am asked why. Why do I like to race? Why do I suggest my client take up racing? There are a lot of reasons why. Racing provides many fitness, social and motivational benefits. Here are just a few of its many positive influences.

Fitness Gains

Racers, even beginning racers, will run at a greater intensity during races than they do in training runs. Even if you do not intend to run hard, your competitive juices will start flowing and you will run at your best pace. This high intensity training will improve your overall fitness levels and decrease your body fat.

When you begin to enter races on a consistent basis, you will want to improve your race times. To do this, you must include some more intense workouts and speed work in your training. This addition of higher intensity workouts on a regular basis will greatly improve overall fitness levels and help you maintain your healthy weight.

Motivation

Racing will provide you with both short and long term goals. A short-term goal may be to complete your first 5K or improve your 5K time. A long-term goal may be to complete a marathon. Having a goal or race to look forward to and advance towards, will motivate you to make time for your daily workouts.

Social benefits

Races are not only a competition; they are also social events. Runners are, as a whole, a very friendly and healthy group. Running events are a great place to meet new people and make new friends. If you compete in local races on a regular basis, you will see the same people over and over at each race.

There are many running clubs that you may join. These clubs will have weekly workouts and frequent social functions. Check with your local running specialty store for area clubs and organizations.

The Rules of Racing

Road racing has a number of unofficial rules. As a new runner, your first races will be made more enjoyable if you follow these informal and unofficial rules of racing.

Register Early

You can register for races in several ways. You can register on race day at the registration table; at a number of pre-race registration locations; by mail; sometimes over the internet.

You should plan on registering early at a pre-race registration site, by mail or by internet. This will guarantee that you will get a T-shirt and a spot in the race. Some popular races have a limited number of entries. By registering early, you will be guaranteed a spot in the race. You also will not have to worry about registering on race day. Some races will give you a discount for registering early, so check the application carefully.

Arrive Early On Race Day

Plan to arrive at least 45 minutes to an hour early on race day. This will give you time to park, jog to the start and warm-up. You will need approximately 20 minutes to warm-up and stretch before the start of the race. You may also need to make a last trip to the portable toilet. The lines may be long at the toilet, so plan accordingly or you may hear the starting gun while you are in the john.

Pin your starting number to the front of your shirt or shorts. The number must be visible throughout the race. Do not pin the number to the back of your shirt. The number must be visible on the front of your body.

If you are late arriving to the race you may have difficulty getting to the starting line on time and you will not have time for an adequate warm up. You also may not get a T-shirt in your size. Avoid the stress and arrive early. You can use the extra time to warm up, relax and enjoy the company of your fellow runners.

Some of the larger races are timed using a computer chip. This chip will be given to you at registration. The chip is attached to the top of your shoe by lacing into your shoelaces or it may have a Velcro strap that you wrap around your ankle. The computer chip will start timing when you pass over the starting line. It will tally your finishing time when you pass over the finish line. This system works especially well in larger races. If you are far back in the starting pack, it may take you up to a minute or even more just to cross the starting line. When using a chip, you will get your actually time, starting when you pass over the starting line, rather than when the starting gun goes off.

Lining up correctly with faster runners to the front and slower runners progressively further back is critical to insure a safe and efficient start. If slower runners are in front, collisions and falls are possible. Slower runners can also be "pulled along" with the faster runners causing the slower runners to fatigue quickly.

There will be a receptacle near the finish line for collecting timing chips. Do not forget to return your chip in the collection bin. If you don't return it, the organizers will charge you for it.

Line Up In Your Proper Starting Position

The fastest runners will line up at the front of the pack. The slower runners will line up farther back. The walkers line up at the back of the starting pack. This is to ensure a safe and efficient start. Make sure that you follow this procedure. If you are an average or slower runner and you line up in front, you will get trampled. You will also make it difficult for the fast runners to get the good start that they need to compete in the race. If you are a fast runner, make sure you line up towards the front or you will be trying to leap frog over slower runners.

Larger races will sometimes have signs directing you to a certain spot in the starting field, depending upon your estimated pace per mile. Be sure to obey these signs. The start of large races can become very congested and if faster runners are trying to get by slower runners, safety can be compromised. In large races, the first runners in the pack will be running at a sub 5 minutes per mile pace. If you cannot run that pace, do not line up at the front of the pack.

Fluid & Aid Stations

Shorter races, such as 5K's and similar distances, will have one or two water stations. They will usually be set up around the one and two mile points in the race. Medium distance races like 10K's will have three or four water stations, set up about a mile apart. Longer races (Marathons, ultra marathons) will have fluid and aid stations at every other mile marker. Some races have them set up at every mile marker. Short and medium distance races will usually have water only. Longer races will have fluid replacement drinks (sports drinks), water and food.

In shorter races, determine how often you should hydrate by monitoring your body and weather conditions. If it is hot, drink a cup of water at each stop. If the weather is cool and you began the race in a well-hydrated condition, you can probably complete a short race without stopping. In a medium distance race, you should drink a cup of water every 15 minutes, in order to stay properly hydrated. In a long race, drink at each station. Do not wait to drink until you feel thirsty. Your feelings of thirst will lag behind your actual hydration level. If you wait until you feel thirsty, you are already dehydrated. You should drink the sports drink in a long race in order to replenish your body's electrolytes and carbohydrates, which become depleted in a long race. If you feel you are becoming overheated, take a cup of water and pour it over your head. This will help cool down your body.

If your race is going to last less than one hour, drinking plain water is fine. During longer events you should consume a sports drink containing sodium and electrolytes. Drinking large amounts of plain water during long exercise sessions can dilute your blood and cause a condition called hyponatremia. Hyponatremia occurs when the sodium levels in your blood drop to dangerously low levels. This condition can cause gastrointestinal upsets, dizziness, fatigue, confusion, disorientation and in extremely serious cases, even death.

Don't stop at the water station when you are drinking. Grab a cup of fluid from the volunteer and keep moving. If you stop at the station, the other runners will be unable to get to the fluids. If you are new to racing, you should walk while you are drinking. If you try to run and drink, you will probably spill more than you take in. Practice pinching the top of the cup together and drinking through the small opening. With practice you will be able to run and drink at the same time. When you are done drinking you can just toss the cup down. The volunteers will pick them up and properly discard them. If there is a trash can within reach, try to toss it in the can, it will help out the overworked volunteers.

Finishing

As you approach the finish line, make sure your number is visible on the front of your shirt or shorts. If your number is not visible you may not be scored and timed properly at the finish. Pass through the finishing chute that you are directed to and keep moving. Do not stop in the chute. There may be a lot of runners finishing at the same time and if the chute becomes blocked a real log-jam can occur. Most races are timed by using a tab that is torn off at the finish. Start tearing your tag off as soon as you pass over the finish line and hand it to the volunteer at the end of the chute. If the race is being timed with the computer chips, just pass through without stopping. There will be a receptacle for you to return your chip near the finish line.

There will be a lot of spectators cheering you on to your finish, so look your best at the finish. Try to put on a burst of speed and give the spectators a wave of acknowledgment. They will appreciate it.

T-shirts

Even if you are new to racing, you don't want to look like it. One thing that makes a new racer stand out is by wearing the race T-shirt that you were given at registration. This is one of those unofficial "un-cool" things that only experienced runners know about. You never wear your race shirt in the race. Wear a shirt from a different race or from the same race at an earlier year. Do that and no one will know that you are a novice racer.

One last comment. The race would not be possible without the generous support of the many volunteers. Be sure to thank them whenever possible. They will greatly appreciate it.

YOUR FIRST 5K

Your first race will be exciting and memorable experience. It can also be the cause of some anxiety. Since you are a new runner, the racing is like a jump into the unknown. You may be nervous about how you are going to do or you may be a bit worried about finishing the race. It is understandable to be apprehensive about your upcoming race. But, put your mind at ease. With proper training you will build the confidence and fitness necessary to comfortably finish your first race. Trust your training. Follow this first 5K training program and your success will be ensured.

Choosing a Race

For your first race, I would suggest a 5K. 5K stands for 5 kilometers which equals 3.1 miles. A 5K is a good choice for a first race because of its relatively short distance and because it is the most common race distance. You should have no trouble finding a 5K race in your area at most times of the year.

You can race at any time of the year, but for your first

one you may want to consider a race in the spring or fall, when the temperatures are mild. Hot or cold weather will make things just a little more difficult. Try to pick a large race for your first one. A larger field will provide a "party atmosphere" that will help motivate and encourage you. A large field will also make new runners less self conscious about where they finish. The large field will provide plenty of runners in the front, middle and back of the pack.

4 Week Training Program For Your First 5K

This is a 4-week program that designed to prepare you for your first race with minimal training. This program will allow you comfortably finish a 5K. It is not intended to run a fast 5K or to improve your speed. You should be able to run comfortably for 2 miles before starting this program. If you have not run before, complete the 8-week beginners program before starting this program.

This program is general in nature. Feel free to make adjustments in order to accommodate scheduling conflicts and individual goals and rate of improvement.

The Workouts

All workouts in this plan are easy runs. Easy runs should be run at a pace that feels fairly comfortable. You should be breathing hard, but should be able to carry on a conversation. If you are breathing so hard that you cannot talk, you are running to hard. If you can sing, you are running to easily.

On the days calling for rest or cross training, you can rest totally or do some cross training. Cross training can be any activity other than running. You could go for a walk, swim, bicycle or do nothing. It is up to you.

Week 1 - Your First 5K Training Schedule

Day	Workout	Comments
Day 1	Rest	Rest
Day 2	Run 2 miles or 3.2 kilometers	Run 2 miles or 3.2 kilometers at an easy pace.
Day 3	Run 2.25 miles or 3.6 kilometers	Run 2.25 miles or 3.6 kilometers at an easy pace
Day 4	Rest or cross train	Rest or cross train. Your cross training activity can be anything physical activity that you enjoy.
Day 5	Run 2 miles or 3.2 kilometers	Run 2 miles or 3.2 kilometers at an easy pace
Day 6	Run 2.25 miles or 3.6 kilometers	Run 2.25 miles or 3.6 kilometers at an easy pace
Day 7	Run 2.5 miles or 4 kilometers	Run 2.5 miles or 4 kilometers at an easy pace

Week 2 - Your First 5K Training Schedule

Day	Workout	Comments
Day 1	Rest	Rest
Day 2	Run 2.5 miles or 4 kilometers	Run 2.5 miles or 4 kilometers at an easy pace
Day 3	Run 2.75 miles or 4.43 kilometers	Run 2.75 miles or 4.43 kilometers at an easy pace.
Day 4	Rest or cross train	Rest or cross train. If you are feeling fatigued take this day completely off. If you are feeling strong go ahead and cross train.
Day 5	Run 2.75 miles or 4.43 kilometers	Run 2.75 miles or 4.43 kilometers at an easy pace
Day 6	Run 2 miles or 3.2 kilometers	Run 2 miles or 3.2 kilometers at an easy pace
Day 7	Run 3 miles or 4.8 kilometers	Run 3 miles or 4.8 kilometers at an easy pace. You are almost running a full 5K distance today. A 5K is 3.1 miles

Week 3 - Your First 5K Training Schedule

Day	Workout	Comments
Day 1	Rest	Rest
Day 2	Run 3 miles or 4.8 kilometers	Run 3 miles or 4.8 kilometers at an easy pace
Day 3	Run 3.25 miles or 5.23 kilometers	Run 3.25 miles or 5.23 kilometers at an easy pace
Day 4	Rest or cross train	Rest or cross train
Day 5	Run 3.25 miles or 5.23 kilometers	Run 3.25 miles or 5.23 kilometers at an easy pace
Day 6	Run 3 or miles or 4.8 kilometers	Run 3 miles or 4.8 kilometers at an easy pace
Day 7	Run 3.5 miles or 5.6 kilometers	Run 3.5 miles or 5.6 kilometers at an easy pace.

Week 4 - Your First 5K Training Schedule

Day	Workout	Comments
Day 1	Rest	Rest
Day 2	Run 3.5 miles or 5.6 kilometers	Run 3.5 miles or 5.6 kilometers at an easy pace
Day 3	Run 3.75 miles or 6 kilometers	Run 3.75 miles or 6 kilometers at an easy pace
Day 4	Rest	Rest
Day 5	Run 3 miles or 4.8 kilometers	Run 3 miles or 4.8 kilometers at an easy pace
Day 6	Rest	Rest
Day 7	Race Day - 3.1 miles or 5K	Enjoy your race!

Finish a 10K

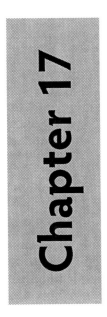

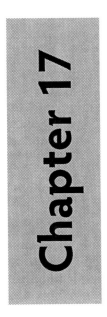**Chapter 17**

If you have completed the beginners program and have finished your first 5K, the next progressive step in your program is to train for and complete your first 10K race. There is no reason you need to do this, but the longer distance of the 10K will further improve your fitness and provide a new and challenging goal. A 10K is twice the distance of your first 5K race or 6.2 miles. Assuming that you are now able to run at least 2 miles comfortably you can train to run a 10K quite easily in just 8 weeks. Those of you that have completed one or more 5K races can start this program on week 2 or 3 and be ready for your 10K in about 6 or 7 weeks.

8 Week Training Program For Your First 10K

This is an 8-week program that designed to prepare you for your first 10K race. This program will allow you comfort-

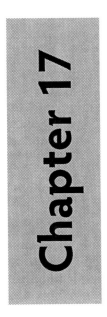

ably finish a 10K. It is not intended to run a fast 10K or to improve your speed. You should be able to run comfortably for 2 miles before starting this program. If you have not run before, complete the 8-week beginners program before starting this program.

This program is general in nature. Feel free to make adjustments in order to accommodate scheduling conflicts and individual goals and rate of improvement.

The Workouts

All workouts in this plan are easy runs. Easy runs should be run at a comfortable pace. Your rate of breathing should be elevated but you should not be out of breath. You should be able to carry on a conversation. If you are breathing so hard that you cannot talk, you are running to hard. If you can sing, you are running to easily.

On the days calling for rest or cross training, you can rest totally or do some cross training. Cross training can be any activity other than running. You could go for a walk, swim, bicycle or do nothing. It is up to you.

Week 1 - Finish a 10K Training Schedule

Day	Workout	Comments
Day 1	Rest	Rest
Day 2	Run 2 miles or 3.2 kilometers	Run 2 miles or 3.2 kilometers at an easy pace. Remember that your easy pace should feel fairly easy. You should be able to sing, but not talk.
Day 3	Run 2.25 miles or 3.6 kilometers	Run 2.25 miles or 3.6 kilometers at an easy pace
Day 4	Rest or cross train	Rest or cross train. Your cross training activity can be any physical activity.
Day 5	Run 2 miles or 3.2 kilometers	Run 2 miles or 3.2 kilometers at an easy pace
Day 6	Run 2.5 miles or 4 kilometers	Run 2.5 miles or 4 kilometers at an easy pace
Day 7	Run 2.75 miles or 4.4 kilometers	Run 2.75 miles or 4.4 kilometers at an easy pace

Week 2 - Finish a 10K Training Schedule

Day	Workout	Comments
Day 1	Rest	Rest
Day 2	Run 2.5 miles or 4 kilometers	Run 2.5 miles or 4 kilometers at an easy pace
Day 3	Run 2.75 miles or 4.4 kilometers	Run 2.75 miles or 4.4 kilometers at an easy pace.
Day 4	Rest or cross train	Rest or cross train. If you are feeling fatigued take this day completely off. If you are feeling strong go ahead and cross train.
Day 5	Run 3 miles or 4.8 kilometers	Run 3 miles or 4.8 kilometers at an easy pace
Day 6	Run 2 miles or 3.2 kilometers	Run 2 miles or 3.2 kilometers at an easy pace
Day 7	Run 3.5 miles or 5.6 kilometers	Run 3.5 miles or 5.6 kilometers at an easy pace.

Week 3 - Finish a 10K Training Schedule

Day	Workout	Comments
Day 1	Rest	Rest
Day 2	Run 3 miles or 4.8 kilometers	Run 3 miles or 4.8 kilometers at an easy pace
Day 3	Run 3.5 miles or 5.6 kilometers	Run 3.5 miles or 5.6 kilometers at an easy pace
Day 4	Rest or cross train	Rest or cross train
Day 5	Run 3 miles or 4.8 kilometers	Run 3 miles or 4.8 kilometers at an easy pace
Day 6	Run 3 or miles or 4.8 kilometers	Run 3 miles or 4.8 kilometers at an easy pace
Day 7	Run 4 miles or 6.4 kilometers	Run 4 miles or 6.4 kilometers at an easy pace.

Week 4 - Finish a 10K Training Schedule

Day	Workout	Comments
Day 1	Rest	Rest
Day 2	Run 3.5 miles or 5.6 kilometers	Run 3.5 miles or 5.6 kilometers at an easy pace
Day 3	Run 4 miles or 6.4 kilometers	Run 4 miles or 6.4 kilometers at an easy pace
Day 4	Rest	Rest
Day 5	Run 3 miles or 4.8 kilometers	Run 3 miles or 4.8 kilometers at an easy pace
Day 6	Run 3 miles or 4.8 kilometers	Run 3 miles or 4.8 kilometers at an easy pace.
Day 7	Run 4.5 miles or 7.2 kilometers	Run 4.5 miles or 7.2 kilometers at an easy pace.

Week 5 - Finish a 10K Training Schedule

Day	Workout	Comments
Day 1	Rest	Rest
Day 2	Run 4 miles or 6.4 kilometers	Run 4 miles or 6.4 kilometers at an easy pace.
Day 3	Run 3 miles or 4.8 kilometers	Run 3 miles or 4.83 kilometers at an easy pace.
Day 4	Rest or cross train	Rest or cross train
Day 5	Run 4 miles or 6.4 kilometers	Run 4 miles or 6.4 kilometers at an easy pace
Day 6	Run 3 miles or 4.8 kilometers	Run 3 miles or 4.8 kilometers at an easy pace
Day 7	Run 5 miles or 8 kilometers	Run 5 miles or 8 kilometers at an easy pace

Week 6 - Finish a 10K Training Schedule

Day	Workout	Comments
Day 1	Rest	Rest
Day 2	Run 4 miles or 6.4 kilometers	Run 4 miles or 6.4 kilometers at an easy pace
Day 3	Run 3 miles or 4.8 kilometers	Run 3 miles or 4.8 kilometers at an easy pace.
Day 4	Rest or cross train	Rest or cross train
Day 5	Run 4 miles or 6.4 kilometers	Run 4 miles or 6.4 kilometers at an easy pace.
Day 6	Run 3 miles or 4.8 kilometers	Run 3 miles or 4.8 kilometers at an easy pace
Day 7	Run 5.5 miles or 8.85 kilometers	Run 5.5 miles or 8.85 kilometers at an easy pace.

Week 7 - Finish a 10K Training Schedule

Day	Workout	Comments
Day 1	Rest	Rest
Day 2	Run 5 miles or 8 kilometers	Run 5 miles or 8 kilometers at an easy pace
Day 3	Run 3 miles or 4.8 kilometers	Run 3 miles or 4.8 kilometers at an easy pace
Day 4	Rest or cross train	Rest or cross train
Day 5	Run 4 miles or 6.4 kilometers	Run 4 miles or 6.4 kilometers at an easy pace
Day 6	Run 3 miles or 4.8 kilometers	Run 3 miles or 4.8 kilometers at an easy pace
Day 7	Run 6 miles or 9.7 kilometers	Run 6 miles or 9.7 kilometers at an easy pace

Week 8 - Finish a 10K Training Schedule

Day	Workout	Comments
Day 1	Rest	Rest
Day 2	Run 5 miles or 8 kilometers	Run 5 miles or 8 kilometers at an easy pace
Day 3	Run 6.2 miles or 10 kilometers	Run 6.2 miles or 10 kilometers at an easy pace. You are now running a full 10K and are fully prepared to finish your first 10K race. You will begin to taper your mileage after this workout so that your muscles will be fully recovered for your race.
Day 4	Rest	Total rest. No running or cross training
Day 5	Run 3 miles or 4.8 kilometers	Run 2 miles or 3.2 kilometers at an easy pace.
Day 6	Rest	Complete rest
Day 7	Race Day - 10K	Run and complete your first 10K race. Enjoy your race and congratulations!

Finish a Half Marathon

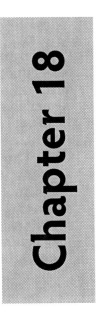

The half marathon is becoming more and more popular each year. A half marathon is 13.1 miles or just over 21 kilometers. This distance is a great stepping stone to finishing a full marathon. It is also excellent for improving your endurance and fitness levels without the time commitments of training for a full marathon. This race distance is also an excellent training tool. Many experienced marathon runners will race half marathons frequently as both a training tool and a test of their fitness level. Half marathon events are easy to find in most areas. There are a wide range of race types available. Do you want to run a flat half marathon on the road? There are plenty of them. How about a hilly trail half marathon? Those are also easy to find.

12 Week Training Program To Finish a Half Marathon

This is a 12-week program that I designed to prepare you to finish a half marathon. It is not intended to run a fast half marathon or finish in a specific time. You should be able to run comfortably for 6 miles before starting this program. If you have not run before, complete the 8-week beginners program and the first 10K program before starting this program. This program is general in nature. Feel free to make adjustments in order to accommodate scheduling conflicts and individual goals and rate of improvement.

This training schedule calls for six workouts per week. I believe that running six days per week with one rest day is the most efficient way to train. It also meets the all important training rule of consistency. The more consistent you are with your training, the better runner you will become. If you would prefer to run only 4 or 5 days per week you can still use this schedule. Take off the easy days number 3 and/or number 6.

The Workouts

All workouts in this plan are easy runs. Easy runs should be run at a comfortable pace. You should be breathing heavily, but should be able to carry on a conversation. If you are breathing so hard that you cannot talk, you are running too hard. If you can sing, you are running too easily.

On the days calling for rest or cross training, you can rest totally or do some cross training. Cross training can be any activity other than running. You could go for a walk, swim, bicycle or do nothing. It is up to you.

The most critical workout in this program is your long run on day 7. You will progress from a 6 mile long run during week 1 to a 15 mile long run on week 11. I like to extend your long run to 15 miles to give you the fitness and confidence to easily finish your half marathon. The 15 mile run will be your longest run. You will taper for 2 weeks before your race. Now - let's get started!

This program has your long run scheduled on day 7. If you would prefer to do your long run on a different day, that is no problem. Just make sure you schedule an easy or rest day before and after your long run.

You can rearrange the sequence in any way that you wish as long as you follow the recommended hard/easy progression. You should always try to avoid doing two hard or long workouts on consecutive days. You will perform better if your body has a chance to rest and recovery between hard efforts.

Week 1 - Finish a Half Marathon Schedule		
Day	Workout	Comments
Day 1	Rest	Rest
Day 2	Run 4 miles or 6.4 kilometers	Run 4 miles or 6.4 kilometers at an easy pace. Remember that your easy pace should feel fairly easy. You should be able to sing, but not talk.
Day 3	Run 3 miles or 4.8 kilometers	Run 3 miles or 4.8 kilometers at an easy pace.
Day 4	Rest or cross train	Rest or cross train. Your cross training activity can be anything physical activity that you enjoy.
Day 5	Run 4 miles or 6.4 kilometers	Run 4 miles or 6.4 kilometers at an easy pace
Day 6	Run 3 miles or 4.8 kilometers	Run 3 miles or 4.8 kilometers at an easy pace
Day7	Run 6 miles or 9.7 kilometers	Run 6 miles or 9.7 kilometers at an easy pace

Week 2 - Finish a Half Marathon Schedule

Day	Workout	Comments
Day 1	Rest	Rest
Day 2	Run 4 miles or 6.4 kilometers	Run 4 miles or 6.4 kilometers at an easy pace
Day 3	Run 3 miles or 4.8 kilometers	Run 3 miles or 4.8 kilometers at an easy pace.
Day 4	Rest or cross train	Rest or cross train. If you are feeling fatigued take this day completely off. If you are feeling strong go ahead and cross train, but try to pick an activity that does not require large amounts of running
Day 5	Run 5 miles or 8 kilometers	Run 5 miles or 8 kilometers at an easy pace
Day 6	Run 3 miles or 4.8 kilometers	Run 3 miles or 4.8 kilometers at an easy pace
Day 7	Run 7 miles or 11.25 kilometers	Run 7 miles or 11.25 kilometers at an easy pace.

Week 3 - Finish a Half Marathon Schedule

Day	Workout	Comments
Day 1	Rest	Rest
Day 2	Run 4 miles or 6.4 kilometers	Run 4 miles or 6.4 kilometers at an easy pace
Day 3	Run 3 miles or 4.8 kilometers	Run 3 miles or 4.8 kilometers at an easy pace
Day 4	Rest or cross train	Rest or cross train
Day 5	Run 5 miles or 8 kilometers	Run 5 miles or 8 kilometers at an easy pace
Day 6	Run 3 or miles or 4.8 kilometers	Run 3 miles or 4.8 kilometers at an easy pace
Day 7	Run 8 miles or 12.87 kilometers	Run 8 miles or 12.87 kilometers at an easy pace.

Week 4 - Finish a Half Marathon Schedule

Day	Workout	Comments
Day 1	Rest	Rest
Day 2	Run 5 miles or 8 kilometers	Run 5 miles or 8 kilometers at an easy pace
Day 3	Run 3 miles or 4.8 kilometers	Run 3 miles or 4.8 kilometers at an easy pace
Day 4	Rest	Rest
Day 5	Run 5 miles or 8 kilometers	Run 5 miles or 8 kilometers at an easy pace
Day 6	Run 3 miles or 4.8 kilometers	Run 3 miles or 4.8 kilometers at an easy pace.
Day 7	Run 9 miles or 14.48 kilometers	Run 9 miles or 14.48 kilometers at an easy pace.

Week 5 - Finish a Half Marathon Schedule

Day	Workout	Comments
Day 1	Rest	Rest
Day 2	Run 4 miles or 6.4 kilometers	Run 4 miles or 6.4 kilometers at an easy pace.
Day 3	Run 3 miles or 4.8 kilometers	Run 3 miles or 4.83 kilometers at an easy pace.
Day 4	Rest or cross train	Rest or cross train
Day 5	Run 4 miles or 6.4 kilometers	Run 4 miles or 6.4 kilometers at an easy pace
Day 6	Run 3 miles or 4.8 kilometers	Run 3 miles or 4.8 kilometers at an easy pace
Day 7	Run 10 miles or 16.1 kilometers	Run 10 miles or 16.1 kilometers at an easy pace

Week 6 - Finish a Half Marathon Schedule

Day	Workout	Comments
Day 1	Rest	Rest
Day 2	Run 5 miles or 8 kilometers	Run 5 miles or 8 kilometers at an easy pace
Day 3	Run 3 miles or 4.8 kilometers	Run 3 miles or 4.8 kilometers at an easy pace.
Day 4	Rest or cross train	Rest or cross train
Day 5	Run 5 miles or 8 kilometers	Run 5 miles or 8 kilometers at an easy pace.
Day 6	Run 3 miles or 4.8 kilometers	Run 3 miles or 4.8 kilometers at an easy pace
Day 7	Run 11 miles or 17.7 kilometers	Run 11 miles or 17.7 kilometers at an easy pace.

Week 7 - Finish a Half Marathon Schedule

Day	Workout	Comments
Day 1	Rest	Rest
Day 2	Run 4 miles or 6.4 kilometers	Run 4 miles or 6.4 kilometers at an easy pace
Day 3	Run 3 miles or 4.8 kilometers	Run 3 miles or 4.8 kilometers at an easy pace
Day 4	Rest or cross train	Rest or cross train
Day 5	Run 4 miles or 6.4 kilometers	Run 4 miles or 6.4 kilometers at an easy pace
Day 6	Run 3 miles or 4.8 kilometers	Run 3 miles or 4.8 kilometers at an easy pace
Day 7	Run 8 miles or 12.87 kilometers	Run 8 miles or 12.87 kilometers at an easy pace

Week 8 - Finish a Half Marathon Schedule

Day	Workout	Comments
Day 1	Rest	Rest
Day 2	Run 5 miles or 8 kilometers	Run 5 miles or 8 kilometers at an easy pace
Day 3	Run 3 miles or 4.8 kilometers	Run 3 miles or 4.8 kilometers at an easy pace
Day 4	Rest or cross train	Rest or cross train
Day 5	Run 6 miles or 9.7 kilometers	Run 6 miles or 9.7 kilometers at an easy pace.
Day 6	Rest	Run 3 miles or 4.8 kilometers at an easy pace
Day 7	Run 13 miles or 21 kilometers	Run 13 miles or 21 kilometers at an easy pace

Week 9 - Finish a Half Marathon Schedule

Day	Workout	Comments
Day 1	Rest	Rest
Day 2	Run 4 miles or 6.4 kilometers	Run 4 miles or 6.4 kilometers at an easy pace
Day 3	Run 3 miles or 4.8 kilometers	Run 3 miles or 4.8 kilometers at an easy pace
Day 4	Rest or cross train	Rest or cross train
Day 5	Run 4 miles or 6.4 kilometers	Run 4 miles or 6.4 kilometers at an easy pace.
Day 6	Run 3 miles or 4.8 kilometers	Run 3 miles or 4.8 kilometers at an easy pace
Day 7	Run 8 miles or 12.87 kilometers	Run 8 miles or 12.87 kilometers at an easy pace

Week 10 - Finish a Half Marathon Schedule

Day	Workout	Comments
Day 1	Rest	Rest
Day 2	Run 5 miles or 8 kilometers	Run 5 miles or 8 kilometers at an easy pace
Day 3	Run 3 miles or 4.8 kilometers	Run 3 miles or 4.8 kilometers at an easy pace
Day 4	Rest or cross train	Rest or cross train
Day 5	Run 6 miles or 9.7 kilometers	Run 6 miles or 9.7 kilometers at an easy pace
Day 6	Run 3 miles or 4.8 kilometers	Run 3 miles or 4.8 kilometers at an easy pace
Day 7	Run 15 miles or 24.14 kilometers	Run 15 miles or 24.14 kilometers at an easy pace

Week 11 - Finish a Half Marathon Schedule

Day	Workout	Comments
Day 1	Rest	Rest
Day 2	Run 4 miles or 6.4 kilometers	Run 4 miles or 6.4 kilometers at an easy pace
Day 3	Run 3 miles or 4.8 kilometers	Run 3 miles or 4.8 kilometers at an easy pace
Day 4	Rest or cross train	Rest or cross train
Day 5	Run 6 miles or 9.7 kilometers	Run 6 miles or 9.7 kilometers at an easy pace
Day 6	Run 3 miles or 4.8 kilometers	Run 3 miles or 4.8 kilometers at an easy pace
Day 7	Run 10 miles or 16.1 kilometers	Run 10 miles or 16.1 kilometers at an easy pace.

Week 12 - Finish a Half Marathon Schedule

Day	Workout	Comments
Day 1	Rest	Rest
Day 2	Run 4 miles or 6.4 kilometers	Run 4 miles or 6.4 kilometers at an easy pace
Day 3	Run 6 miles or 9.7 kilometers	Run 6 miles or 9.7 kilometers at an easy pace.
Day 4	Rest	Complete rest. No running or cross training
Day 5	Rest	Complete rest
Day 6	Rest	Complete rest
Day 7	Race Day - 13.1 miles	Finish your half marathon - Enjoy and congratulations!

Congratulations on finishing your half marathon. Pat yourself on the back and take a few days off to recovery. You deserve it! Are you ready to take the next step of finishing a full marathon? While the marathon is not for everyone, it is the ultimate goal of many runners and you are very close to doing it. You are half way there already.

Finish a Marathon

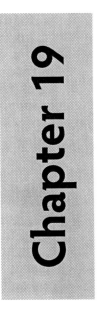

At one time only highly experienced runners attempted to run a marathon. Today things are very different. Runners of all abilities and experience levels are successfully finishing this challenging but exhilarating distance. There are an almost endless number of reasons athletes have for running a marathon. For some it is a life changing event. Some run it to honor a friend or family member. Some do it to change their life. Others run for fun or competition. Whatever your reason, your first marathon will be an occasion that you will remember for your entire life.

16 Week Beginning Marathon Program

This is a 16-week program that I designed to prepare you to finish a full marathon. This program will allow you finish, but not race a marathon. It is not intended to prepare you to compete for top positions or finish in a specific time. You should be able to run comfortably for 6 miles before starting this program. If you have not run before, complete the 8-week beginners program and the finish a 10K schedule before starting this program. Just as the other training schedules in this book, feel free to make adjustments in order to accommodate scheduling conflicts and individual goals and rate of improvement.

If you have just finished the half marathon training program you are ready to jump into this full marathon program at week 5. You will be prepared to run your first marathon in just 12 weeks.

The Workouts

This training schedule is designed to prepare you to finish a marathon. It is not intended to improve your speed or train you to finish in a specific time. Since the goal of this program is to finish the race the workouts concentrate on building your endurance and strength. All workouts are performed at an easy pace. Remember that when you are running at an easy pace you should be able to speak clearly but you should not be able to sing.

Many beginning marathon programs suggest using frequent walking breaks. That is a good strategy and you can use walking breaks in this program also. Just keep in mind that your training should mimic your race goal as closely as possible. If you plan on using walking breaks in your marathon go ahead and use similar walking breaks during your training. Some beginning runners set a goal of running the entire marathon. If that is your goal, you should train the same way, without walking breaks. Training is like practicing any other skill. If you practice using walking breaks, that is what you are preparing your body to do. If you want to complete the marathon without walking, then you should train the same way - without walking breaks.

Week 1

For your first week of marathon training you will start with a long run of 6 miles. You should already be comfortable with a 6 mile run at this point. Throughout this training schedule you will be gradually, but steadily increasing the distance of your long run. Your long run is the keystone workout of this training schedule. Since your goal in your first marathon is just to finish, your long run is the workout that will get you there. It will build your cardiovascular endurance, muscular endurance and mental toughness. In later marathon programs when you want to improve your pace you will be doing other types of workouts to increase your speed and speed endurance. For now it is best just to concentrate on building your base of endurance.

Week 1 - Finish a Marathon Schedule		
Day	Workout	Comments
Day 1	Rest	Rest
Day 2	4 miles or 6 kilometers	Run 4 miles or 6 kilometers at an easy pace. Remember that your easy pace should feel fairly easy. You should be able to sing, but not talk.
Day 3	3 miles or 5 kilometers	Run 3 miles or 5 kilometers at an easy pace.
Day 4	Rest or cross train	Rest or cross train. Your cross training activity can be anything physical activity that you enjoy.
Day 5	4 miles or 6 kilometers	Run 4 miles or 6 kilometers at an easy pace
Day 6	3 miles or 5 kilometers	Run 3 miles or 5 kilometers at an easy pace
Day 7	6 miles or 10 kilometers	Run 6 miles or 10 kilometers at an easy pace

Week 2

You have completed your first full week of marathon training. Great job! Consistency is a very important part of any running program and is even more critical when it comes to marathon training. Make sure you commit yourself completely to your training. The marathon is a difficult event that can become a monster if you don't complete the required training. Stay with it and you will succeed.

This week your long run will be extended to 8 miles or about 13 kilometers. If you are planning on completing the marathon using a run/walk combination go ahead and take similar walking breaks during your training. If you want to run the entire marathon, do not take walking breaks during training.

Week 2 - Finish a Marathon Schedule		
Day	Workout	Comments
Day 1	Rest	Rest
Day 2	4 miles or 6 kilometers	Run 4 miles or 6 kilometers at an easy pace
Day 3	3 miles or 4.8 kilometers	Run 3 miles or 5 kilometers at an easy pace.
Day 4	Rest or cross train	Rest or cross train. If you are feeling fatigued take this day completely off. If you are feeling strong go ahead and cross train, but try to pick an activity that does not require large amounts of running
Day 5	5 miles or 8 kilometers	Run 5 miles or 8 kilometers at an easy pace
Day 6	3 miles or 4.8 kilometers	Run 3 miles or 5 kilometers at an easy pace
Day 7	8 miles or 13 kilometers	Run 8 miles or 13 kilometers at an easy pace.

Week 3

Rest is an important part of your training schedule. You have two scheduled rest days during each training week. That should be enough allow your body to recover from the training. Avoid the temptation to run on your rest days. At the beginning level your body needs those days off to stay strong and healthy. Running is a sport in which the benefits build up year after year. As your body gets fitter you will be able to run more days per week without suffering from over training or over reaching syndromes. But as a beginning runner you really need at least one and preferable two complete rest days per week. When training for shorter races, one rest day per week is usually enough. I prefer two rest days per week when training for your first marathon.

This week your long run is up to 10 miles or about 16 kilometers. Your long runs may start to feel difficult towards the end of your workout. Stay strong and keep going. This is what training is all about.

Week 3 - Finish a Marathon Schedule		
Day	Workout	Comments
Day 1	Rest	Rest
Day 2	4 miles or 6.4 kilometers	Run 4 miles or 6 kilometers at an easy pace
Day 3	3 miles or 4.8 kilometers	Run 3 miles or 5 kilometers at an easy pace
Day 4	Rest or cross train	Rest or cross train
Day 5	5 miles or 8 kilometers	Run 5 miles or 8 kilometers at an easy pace
Day 6	3 or miles or 4.8 kilometers	Run 3 miles or 5 kilometers at an easy pace
Day 7	10 miles or 16.1 kilometers	Run 10 miles or 16 kilometers at an easy pace.

Week 4

Marathon training is a mental challenge as well as a physical one. You are doing something that your mind is probably telling you not to do. Remember that you are in control. You have the ability to over ride any negative thoughts or emotions that your mind tries to throw at you. Always stay positive. When you start to fatigue and struggle during long runs or any other part of your training, replace negative self talk with positive. Instead of saying "I am getting really tired and I can't do this" - say "I am starting to feel fatigue, but I know that is a normal part of marathon training. I am strong enough to fight through this and finish my workout." When you think positive thoughts your body will soon follow suit.

Week 4 - Finish a Marathon Schedule		
Day	Workout	Comments
Day 1	Rest	Rest - Rest days are important. Ignore the desire to run on your days off.
Day 2	5 miles or 8 kilometers	Run 5 miles or 8 kilometers at an easy pace
Day 3	3 miles or 5 kilometers	Run 3 miles or 5 kilometers at an easy pace
Day 4	Rest	Rest
Day 5	5 miles or 8 kilometers	Run 5 miles or 8 kilometers at an easy pace
Day 6	3 miles or 5 kilometers	Run 3 miles or 5 kilometers at an easy pace.
Day 7	12 miles or 19 kilometers	Run 12 miles or 19 kilometers at an easy pace.

Week 5

You have hit a milestone this week. Your long run of 14 miles or about 22 kilometers is over half of the distance of your marathon. You are over half way there! If you are taking walking breaks in your race, keep taking the walking breaks during training. The day after your long run is always a scheduled rest day. Don't cross train on that day. You need complete rest to recover from the effects of your long run. This becomes critical after this week as your long runs become longer and more difficult.

Week 5 - Finish a Marathon Schedule		
Day	Workout	Comments
Day 1	Rest	Rest
Day 2	4 miles or 6 kilometers	Run 4 miles or 6 kilometers at an easy pace.
Day 3	3 miles or 5 kilometers	Run 3 miles or 5 kilometers at an easy pace.
Day 4	Rest or cross train	Rest or cross train. Swimming and bicycling are both very good cross training activities.
Day 5	4 miles or 6 kilometers	Run 4 miles or 6 kilometers at an easy pace
Day 6	3 miles or 5 kilometers	Run 3 miles or 5 kilometers at an easy pace
Day 7	14 miles or 22 kilometers	Run 14 miles or 22 kilometers at an easy pace

Week 6

For the first 5 weeks of this schedule you increased the distance of your long run each week. Starting with this week you will be doing a long run every other week instead of each week. Once you reach 12 to 14 miles your body need an extra week of recovery time in order to fully rest, restore and strengthen itself so that you stay strong. Doing a long run each week at this level could result in over training problems such as chronic fatigue, weak muscles, depression, lack of motivation, poor performance and frequent infections.

Week 6 - Finish a Marathon Schedule		
Day	Workout	Comments
Day 1	Rest	Rest
Day 2	5 miles or 8 kilometers	Run 5 miles or 8 kilometers at an easy pace
Day 3	3 miles or 5 kilometers	Run 3 miles or 5 kilometers at an easy pace.
Day 4	Rest or cross train	Rest or cross train
Day 5	5 miles or 8 kilometers	Run 5 miles or 8 kilometers at an easy pace.
Day 6	3 miles or 5 kilometers	Run 3 miles or 5 kilometers at an easy pace
Day 7	8 miles or 13 kilometers	Run 8 miles or 13 kilometers at an easy pace. You will start doing a long run on every other week from now on.

Week 7

Drinking on the run is a skill that must be learned and practiced. If you are planning a marathon with walking breaks you should walk all of the fluid stations in the marathon. That way you will easily get down all of your fluids. If you are planning on running the entire distance, including the fluid stations, you need to learn to drink on the run. The fluids will be handed to you, by a race volunteer, in a paper cup. Take the cup carefully and try not to spill most of it. Immediately pinch the top of the cup nearly closed to avoid further spilling. Drink through the pinched top. It takes some practice but eventually you will be able to get most of the fluid down with minimal spilling. By the end of the race you should be an expert hydrator.

Week 7 - Finish a Marathon Schedule		
Day	Workout	Comments
Day 1	Rest	Rest
Day 2	4 miles or 6 kilometers	Run 4 miles or 6 kilometers at an easy pace
Day 3	3 miles or 5 kilometers	Run 3 miles or 5 kilometers at an easy pace
Day 4	Rest or cross train	Rest or cross train. The decision whether to cross train or rest totally is up to you. If you are feeling fatigued take the day completely off. If you feel strong you may cross train or rest.
Day 5	4 miles or 6 kilometers	Run 4 miles or 6 kilometers at an easy pace
Day 6	3 miles or 5 kilometers	Run 3 miles or 5 kilometers at an easy pace
Day 7	16 miles or 26 kilometers	Run 16 miles or 26 kilometers at an easy pace

Week 8

You hit another major milestone in your training this week. This is the half way point in your training schedule. You are probably feeling strong at this point. You are gaining fitness, endurance and strength. Even though you are getting stronger your long runs are most likely getting tougher. That is normal. During each long run you are challenging your self further. That is what training is all about. You challenge your body and it responds by becoming stronger. Keep at it and stay positive. You are half way there and you are going to make it all the way.

This weeks schedule includes an extra day of rest. Your body need some extra recovery time after the first 8 weeks of training. I would prefer total rest on your extra recovery day, but if you would like to do some cross training that would also be OK.

Week 8 - Finish a Marathon Schedule		
Day	Workout	Comments
Day 1	Rest	Rest
Day 2	5 miles or 8 kilometers	Run 5 miles or 8 kilometers at an easy pace
Day 3	3 miles or 5 kilometers	Run 3 miles or 5 kilometers at an easy pace
Day 4	Rest or cross train	Rest or cross train
Day 5	6 miles or 10 kilometers	Run 6 miles or 10 kilometers at an easy pace.
Day 6	Rest	Rest - You have an extra day of rest this week. This will help your body recover from the first 8 weeks of hard training.
Day 7	10 miles or 16 kilometers	Run 10 miles or 16 kilometers at an easy pace

Week 9

Staying properly hydrated is very important when you are running long distances. During shorter distances you can drink plain water. During long training runs and during your race you should consume a sports drink containing sodium and other electrolytes. You lose a lot of sodium and other essential minerals in your sweat when you are running. Those mineral losses cause a drop in your blood sodium levels. If you hydrate with plain water you dilute the sodium levels in your blood ever further. That can result in a dangerous condition called hyponatremia. To avoid that always drinks a sports drink during long training runs and at each fluid station during your marathon.

You will continue to extend your long this week. You will be doing an 18 mile or 29 kilometer run on day 7.

Week 9 - Finish a Marathon Schedule		
Day	Workout	Comments
Day 1	Rest	Rest
Day 2	4 miles or 6 kilometers	Run 4 miles or 6 kilometers at an easy pace
Day 3	3 miles or 5 kilometers	Run 3 miles or 5 kilometers at an easy pace
Day 4	Rest or cross train	Rest or cross train
Day 5	4 miles or 6 kilometers	Run 4 miles or 6 kilometers at an easy pace.
Day 6	3 miles or 5 kilometers	Run 3 miles or 5 kilometers at an easy pace
Day 7	18 miles or 29 kilometers	Run 18 miles or 29 kilometers at an easy pace

Week 10

I strongly suggest incorporating strength training into your training program. Hopefully you have been doing the suggested strength training since you started with the beginners program. Strength training builds up a base of fitness that will improve your overall fitness, build up strength in your lower body to support your training runs and help you avoid injury. Stronger leg muscles can make a big difference in the quality of your marathon training and your performance in your race. You should perform strength training on a year round basis.

Week 10 - Finish a Marathon Schedule		
Day	Workout	Comments
Day 1	Rest	Rest
Day 2	5 miles or 8 kilometers	Run 5 miles or 8 kilometers at an easy pace
Day 3	3 miles or 5 kilometers	Run 3 miles or 5 kilometers at an easy pace
Day 4	Rest or cross train	Rest or cross train
Day 5	6 miles or 10 kilometers	Run 6 miles or 10 kilometers at an easy pace
Day 6	3 miles or 5 kilometers	Run 3 miles or 5 kilometers at an easy pace
Day 7	8 miles or 13 kilometers	Run 8 miles or 13 kilometers at an easy pace

Week 11

This week your long run is up to 20 miles or 32 kilometers. Many popular marathon training programs only extend your long run to 20 miles before starting to taper. I disagree with that practice. Twenty miles leaves you 6.2 miles or a full 10K that you have not properly prepared your body for. Another way to look at it is that you have only trained for 75% of the full distance. Limiting your long run to a maximum of 20 miles can cause the last 6.2 miles to be very difficult and relatively painful. This training schedule will extend your long run another 2 miles. That give you only 4.2 miles to complete in your marathon. That is a more manageable distance. Later, in more advanced marathon programs, I would suggest extending your long run even farther to 24 or more miles.

Week 11 - Finish a Marathon Schedule		
Day	Workout	Comments
Day 1	Rest	Rest
Day 2	4 miles or 6 kilometers	Run 4 miles or 6 kilometers at an easy pace
Day 3	3 miles or 5 kilometers	Run 3 miles or 5 kilometers at an easy pace
Day 4	Rest or cross train	Rest or cross train
Day 5	6 miles or 10 kilometers	Run 6 miles or 10 kilometers at an easy pace
Day 6	3 miles or 5 kilometers	Run 3 miles or 5 kilometers at an easy pace
Day 7	20 miles or 32 kilometers	Run 20 miles or 32 kilometers at an easy pace.

Week 12

A proper marathon diet is a bit different than a normal healthy diet. What you should eat depends upon what you are doing at the time. During your marathon training you will always need more carbohydrates than you normally do. Carbohydrates are the preferred fuel for generating the energy required for running or any other activity. You need between 8 and 10 grams of carbohydrates per pound of body weight to properly fuel your marathon training. Most of the time you should try to eat mostly complex carbohydrates. There is an exception to that rule. When you are running your marathon you want the energy from carbohydrates to get to your muscles as quickly as possible. In that case you should eat simple carbohydrates because they enter your bloodstream and get to your muscles much faster than complex carbs.

Day	Workout	Comments
Day 1	Rest	Rest
Day 2	4 miles or 6 kilometers	Run 4 miles or 6 kilometers at an easy pace
Day 3	6 miles or 10 kilometers	Run 6 miles or 10 kilometers at an easy pace.
Day 4	Rest or cross train	Rest or cross train
Day 5	6 miles or 10 kilometers	Run 6 miles or 10 kilometers at an easy pace
Day 6	3 miles or 5 kilometers	Run 3 miles or 5 kilometers at an easy pace
Day 7	8 miles or 13 kilometers	Run 8 miles or 13 kilometers at an easy pace.

Week 12 - Finish a Marathon Schedule

Week 13

This is a big week for you. This week you will be doing the longest run of your training program. Your 22 mile or 35 kilometer run on day 7 will be your longest run and your last true long run of this schedule. After this week you will begin to taper for your race. Make this long run a good one. Stay focused and mentally strong. Keep up a steady pace throughout the run. If you are doing a run/walk combination take your walking breaks only as planned. If you are planning to run the entire marathon, do not take any walking breaks. Stay strong and run through the tough spots. This is not only your last long run but is a rehearsal for your race. Use this opportunity to work on your mental toughness. It will pay off in your marathon.

Week 13 - Finish a Marathon Schedule		
Day	Workout	Comments
Day 1	Rest	Rest
Day 2	4 miles or 6 kilometers	Run 4 miles or 6 kilometers at an easy pace
Day 3	3 miles or 5 kilometers	Run 3 miles or 5 kilometers at an easy pace
Day 4	Rest or cross train	Rest or cross train
Day 5	6 miles or 10 kilometers	Run 6 miles or 10 kilometers at an easy pace
Day 6	3 miles or 5 kilometers	Run 3 miles or 5 kilometers at an easy pace
Day 7	22 miles or 35 kilometers	Run 22 miles or 35 kilometers at an easy pace. This will be your longest run. You will begin to taper after this week.

Week 14

This week you will begin to taper. A taper is a reduction in the quantity of training. Gradually reducing your training volume in the last three weeks leading up to your race is a critical part of your training. The reduced volume will allow your body, muscles and mind a chance to rest, recover and rebuild in strength. You will start your race with your mind and muscles at full strength. Your taper will be gradual. You will see a reduction in daily mileage as well as the introduction of additional rest days. Do not run or extend your mileage thinking it will benefit you in your race. Your hard training is done. Now it is time to allow your muscles to rebuild in strength. Any hard training at this point will be counter productive.

Week 14 - Finish a Marathon Schedule		
Day	Workout	Comments
Day 1	Rest	Rest
Day 2	6 miles or 10 kilometers	Run 6 miles or 10 kilometers at an easy pace
Day 3	3 miles or 5 kilometers	Run 3 miles or 5 kilometers at an easy pace
Day 4	Rest or cross train	Rest or cross train
Day 5	6 miles or 10 kilometers	Run 6 miles or 10 kilometers at an easy pace
Day 6	3 miles or 5 kilometers	Run 3 miles or 5 kilometers at an easy pace
Day 7	10 miles or 16 kilometers	Run 10 miles or 16 kilometers at an easy pace.

Week 15

You are down to your last two weeks of training. You are almost there. Be careful to avoid a mental letdown at this point. Your physical training is winding down but you must stay strong mentally. Be very careful with your diet during these last two weeks. You should be eating a diet that is 65% to 70% carbohydrate. Concentrate on complex carbohydrates such as whole grains, vegetables, beans and legumes. You also need a slightly higher amount of lean proteins to supply the building blocks for your recovering muscles. Eat lean healthy proteins such as chicken, fish, soy protein and skim milk. Avoid high fat food or simple carbohydrates.

Week 15 - Finish a Marathon Schedule		
Day	Workout	Comments
Day 1	Rest	Rest
Day 2	Run 4 miles or 6 kilometers	Run 4 miles or 6 kilometers at an easy pace
Day 3	Run 3 miles or 5 kilometers	Run 3 miles or 5 kilometers at an easy pace
Day 4	Rest	Complete rest. No running or cross training
Day 5	Run 3 miles or 5 kilometers	Run 3 miles or 5 kilometers at an easy pace
Day 6	Rest	Complete rest
Day 7	Run 8 miles or 13 kilometers	Run 8 miles or 13 kilometers at an easy pace

Week 16

You've done it! You are about to finish your final training week for your first marathon. If you have followed the schedule you will succeed in meeting your goal of finishing a marathon. This week has only two workouts. You will rest the final three days before your race. Try to avoid any strenuous non running activity on these rest days.

The evening before your race is a good time to carboload. The traditional way to carbo-load is to eat a pasta dinner. While pasta is traditional there is no physical reason you need to eat pasta. Any meal that is high in complex carbohydrates will get the job done. The purpose of carboloading is to "top off" your body's fuel reserves so that you start the race with a full tank.

On race morning, get up early and eat a light meal composed of mostly complex carbohydrates. Avoid any high fat foods, high fiber foods or simple sugars. Also remember to drink enough fluids early so that you start your marathon fully hydrated. Good luck with your race and congratulations on meeting your goal!

Week 16 - Finish a Marathon Schedule		
Day	Workout	Comments
Day 1	Rest	Complete rest
Day 2	4 miles or 6 kilometers	Run 4 miles or 6 kilometers at an easy pace
Day 3	3 miles or 5 kilometers	Run 3 miles or 5 kilometers at an easy pace
Day 4	Rest	Complete rest
Day 5	Rest	Complete rest
Day 6	Rest	Complete rest
Day 7	Race Day	Finish your marathon. Enjoy and congratulations!

Going Farther and Faster

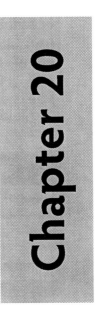

O ne of the many reasons that running is such a great sport is the ability to tailor the activity to your specific goals, needs and desires. Some runners enjoy cruising through their daily run at a nice, relaxed pace. They are running simply to enjoy the many physical and mental benefits of running and exercise. Other runners like to run at a faster pace. They may be training for competitions or they may just love the feeling of challenging their body and minds to overcome physical and mental barriers. Many runners want to run a few miles to reduce stress, maintain their weight or stay fit. Some others like to build their endurance to higher levels with a weekly long run. You can do whatever you want to do and meet any goal you desire.

If part of your goals are to build up your speed and endurance there are a number of specific workouts that will help you get there. You will improve your endurance by simply including a weekly long run in your training program. Increasing your speed is slightly more complicated.

There are six primary components involved in increasing your ability to run farther and faster over long distances. Since this is a beginners manual I will not get too technical or detailed, but it will help if you have a basic understanding of the concepts. The six main components of endurance and distance running speed are:

- **VO₂ max** - This is a measure of the maximum amount of oxygen that you body is able to process. Theoretically, the more oxygen your body can process, the more energy you are able to produce. A higher VO_2 max usually means you are able to run at higher intensities or speeds.

- **vVO₂ max** - Don't let all of these fancy looking terms throw you. This one is really simple. It is your running velocity at your VO_2 max. In other words, how fast you are running when you reach your body's peak oxygen processing capacity. This is a more reliable indicator of how fit you are than VO2 max alone because it factors in all of the other components of running performance.

- **Lactate Turn point** - Remember in the chapter on Your Body in Action, I touched on how lactic acid is produced quicker and in greater amounts when you run faster? Your lactate turn point is the level at which lactic acid begins to be produced faster than your body can process it. When that happens you begin to fatigue and are forced to slow down. You can raise your lactate turn point through proper training. That will allow you to run faster for longer distances.

- **Speed and Neuromuscular Conditioning** - Your brain controls your muscles by sending signals through a system of nerves and nerve receptors in your muscles. High speed training will condition that system and increase your overall speed.

- **Running Economy** - This is a measure of how efficiently you run. A good comparison is the gas mileage of your car. A highly efficient car will get more miles to a gallon of gas. In the same sense, a highly efficient runner will able to run faster and farther using less energy. There are a number of components involved in running economy including lactate turn point, neuromuscular conditioning and running strength.

- **Endurance** - This one is really a no brainer. It is fairly obvious that you need to continue to build up your ability to run long distances to improve as a runner. Improving your endurance builds the strength and stamina of your muscles and connective tissues. Endurance is best built up through the use of long runs.

OK - those are the running systems that you will need to train in order to improve your running speed and performance. There are a number of specific types of workouts you can do that will help train all of those systems. None of these workouts train only one system. Each of the following types of workouts concentrate on one system, but each will contribute something to building each of the various distance running components.

Because of the multiple systems that you need to train to improve as runner you should use a multi-pace training schedule. A multi-pace training program will include all of the various types of workouts on a weekly or biweekly basis, rather than concentrating on one type of workout.

Speed Building Workouts

These workouts are specifically intended to build your VO_2 max, vVO_2 max and neuromuscular conditioning but also contribute to improving your lactate turn point and running economy. If you have been reading other running publications you may have heard these workouts referred to as interval training, speed work or running economy workouts. Because of the very fast pace of speed workouts, they are broken up into short repeats with rest intervals inserted between the work repeats. This is the origin of the term "interval training".

400 Meter Repeats

These are short repeats at are performed at a pace that is at about a rating of 17 to 18 or very hard on the RPE scale. If you have participated in 5K races, your pace should be about 5 to 10 seconds per mile faster than your 5K pace. I would suggest doing this workout on a 400 meter track in your neighborhood. That will make it easy to judge your distance. You can also do this workout on a treadmill. The precision of the treadmill even increases the quality of this type of training run.

After a warm up, run 400 meters at RPE 17 to 18 or just faster than your current 5K race pace. Recover with 400 meters at a very easy pace or rest completely for 2 minutes. Repeat this 4 to 12 times. Start your training with fewer repeats and gradually build up the number of repeats as your fitness level increases.

Time/Distance	Pace	Comments
10 Minutes	Very Easy or Walk	Warm up thoroughly
400 Meters	Very hard pace - 5 to 10 seconds faster than 5K pace	Pace should feel very hard but not maximal
400 Meters or 2 minutes	Very Easy or Complete Rest	Run at an easy pace for 400 meters or rest completely for 2 minutes.
400 Meters	Very hard pace - 5 to 10 seconds faster than 5K pace	Maintain your pace throughout the workout
400 Meters or 2 minutes	Very Easy or Complete Rest	Keep repeating this sequence of 400 meters hard and 400 meters or 2 minutes of rest for your planned number of repeats.

800 Meter Repeats

This is another popular track interval workout that translates very well to the treadmill or the road. After a warm up, run 800 meters at RPE 16 to 17 or a hard to very hard pace. For you racers out there this should be at your current 5K race pace. Then slow down to a very easy pace for 400 meters to recover or rest completely for 2 minutes. Repeat this 2 to 8 times. Start with 2 repetitions early in your training and gradually increase to 8 repetitions as your fitness level increases.

Time/Distance	Pace	Comments
10 Minutes	Very Easy	Always warm up before beginning a hard workout
800 Meters	Hard to Very Hard - 5K Pace	Your pace will feel hard - about 16 to 17 on the RPE
400 Meters or 2 minutes	Very Easy or Walk	Run at an easy pace for 400 meters or rest completely for 2 minutes.
800 Meters	Hard to Very Hard - 5K Pace	Try to maintain a steady pace. Don't let yourself slow down
400 Meters or 2 minutes	Very Easy or Walk	Keep repeating this sequence of 800 meters hard and 400 meters or 2 minutes of rest for your planned number of repeats.

5 x 1, 2 or 3 Minute Repeats

After mastering the 400 meter repeats and the 800 meter repeats you will be ready to move on to 1 minute repeats. These repeats are performed at a faster pace of around RPE 18 to 19 - a very, very hard pace. These are very close to the fastest pace you can maintain for the time of the workout. This is a difficult workout that is very good for developing speed and running economy. It is also very useful for improving your ability to run at near VO$_2$ max pace for long distances.

After a warm up, run one minute at RPE 18 to 19. If you do 5K races this pace is about 15 to 20 seconds per mile faster than your current 5K race pace. Then rest completely for 2 minutes to recover. Repeat this 5 times.

As your fitness level increases, you can increase the distance from 1 minute to 2 minutes and finally to 3 minutes. If you have trouble completing the workout, increase the recovery interval.

Time/Distance	Pace	Comments
10 Minutes	Very Easy	A warm up is very important before any workout
1 Minute	RPE 18 to 19	Try to maintain a consistent hard pace for the entire minute
2 minutes	Total Rest	Complete Rest
1 Minute	RPE 18 to 19	This is a very, very hard pace
2 Minutes	Total Rest	Complete Rest
1 Minute	RPE 18 to 19	Maintain your pace
2 Minutes	Total Rest	Complete Rest - No Jogging
1 Minute	RPE 18 to 19	The fourth and fifth repeat will start to feel very hard. Try to keep up a strong pace
2 Minutes	Total Rest	Complete Rest
1 Minute	RPE 18 to 19	Last One
2 Minutes	Walking	Walk for 2 minutes to cool down

Beginners Ladder

A ladder is a workout in which you increase the pace of your workout like "climbing up a ladder". This is an entry level ladder workout that is appropriate for beginners, but can also be used effectively by all levels. This workout improves your ability to run fast when you are fatigued.

After a warm up of 10 to 15 minutes, run 1 mile at RPE 12 to 13 or a comfortable pace, then speed up to RPE 14 to 15 or a somewhat hard to hard pace for 800 meters. If you have raced a 10K this is right at your 10K race pace. Then speed up again to RPE 16 to 17 or a hard to very hard pace for 400 meters. This is about your 5K pace. There is no recovery between the different paces. Cool down with 10 to 15 minutes of easy running. Start with just one of these ladders. As your fitness level increases you can do two or even three of these short ladders.

Time/Distance	Pace	Comments
10 Minutes	Easy Pace	Warm up for 10 minutes or until you feel loose and warm
1 Mile	Comfortable to Somewhat Hard Pace	You do not take any recovery between the portions of this workout. Just keep climbing the ladder.
800 Meters	Somewhat Hard to Hard Pace - RPE 14 to 15	If you have raced a 10K this portion is right at your 10K race pace.
400 Meters	Hard to Very Hard - 5K Pace	Keep climbing to your hard to very hard pace
5 Minutes	Very Easy	Cool Down

Beginners Pyramid

A pyramid is similar to a ladder workout except that you climb one side of the pyramid and then go back down with no recovery. This is an entry level pyramid workout. Don't try this one until you have become comfortable with the ladder workout.

Warm up for 10 to 15 minutes. Begin your workout by running 3/4 mile or 1200 meters at a comfortable pace. Speed up to RPE 14 to 15 or a somewhat hard to hard pace for 1/2 mile or 800 meters. Again, that is about 10K race pace. Now increase your speed to RPE 16 to 17 or very hard pace (5K pace) for 1/4 mile or 400 Meters

Now travel back down the pyramid by running 800 Meters at a hard or 10K pace and finish with 3/4 mile at a comfortable pace. There is no recovery time between the different paces. Cool down with 10 to 15 minutes of easy running or walking.

Time/Distance	Pace	Comments
10 Minutes	Easy Pace	Warm Up
3/4 Mile or 1200 Meters	Comfortable to Somewhat Hard Pace	This pace is slower than 10K pace but faster than an easy pace
800 Meters	Somewhat Hard to Hard Pace - RPE 14 to 15	Climb the pyramid with no recovery
400 Meters	Hard to Very Hard - 5K Pace	This is the top of your pyramid
800 Meters	Somewhat Hard to Hard Pace - RPE 14 to 15	Now you start back down the pyramid
400 Meters	Hard to Very Hard - 5K Pace	Try to maintain this hard pace for 400 meters
10 Minutes	Very Easy Pace	Cool Down

Speed Endurance Building Workouts

Building speed is only one phase of improving your speed and performance as a distance runner. You not only need the speed but you need to maintain a quality pace over long distances. That is where speed endurance workouts come in. Speed endurance runs have many aliases. They have been called lactate threshold runs, anaerobic conditioning, tempo runs, anaerobic threshold training, sustained runs and steady-state runs. Regardless of what term you use, the goal of these workouts are the same. They are designed to improve the ability of your body to process and produce energy from the lactic acid produced by your running, which will improve your ability to maintain a quality pace over a long distance.

The training paces that are best for building your speed endurance range from RPE 14 to RPE 19. If you have participated in 5K or 10K races that equals a pace of about 10 to 15 seconds per mile slower than your 10K race pace to just faster than your 5K race pace.

Speed Endurance Workouts help build all of your various running systems, but they are primarily intended to improve your lactate turn point. When you raise your lactate turn point you become more efficient at using the lactic acid produced by high intensity running to produce more energy. As you raise your lactate turn point you are able to run at faster paces for longer distances before you become fatigued.

Lactate Turn Point Cruiser

This is a beginners speed endurance workout in which the goal is to maintain a pace that is just below your lactate turn point. Similar workouts have been called cruise intervals, steady-state running and anaerobic threshold runs. This is a key training run that is used for all long distance race training and trains your body to maintain a quality pace for an extended period. This workout also toughens you mentally so that you can keep up a good tempo when fatigued.

After a 5 to 10 minute warm up, run between 15 and 45 minutes at a pace that is about RPE 13 to 14 or somewhat hard. This is about 10 seconds per mile slower than your current 10K race pace or about 25 seconds slower than your 5K race pace. Perform this workout without stopping or slowing for recovery. The idea is to maintain your pace for the entire duration of the workout. Cool down with 5 minutes of easy running.

Time/Distance	Pace	Comments
5 - 10 Minutes	Easy Pace	Warm Up
15 - 40 Minutes	Somewhat hard pace or about RPE 13 - 14. 10 seconds per mile slower that your 10K race pace or 25 seconds per mile slower than your 5K race pace.	Your first workout should be about 15 minutes. Increase your time gradually each time you do this workout, as your fitness level improves
10 Minutes	Easy Pace	Cool Down

One Mile Repeats

One mile repeats are another popular track workout that is a good beginners speed endurance workout. After a warm up, run one mile at RPE 14 to 15 or a somewhat hard to hard pace. This is equal to your current 10K race pace or about 15 second per mile slower than your 5K race pace. Then slow down to a comfortable pace for 1/4 mile to recover before speeding up again to 10K pace for the next segment. You could also recover with complete rest for 2 minutes. Repeat this 2 to 6 times depending upon your experience and fitness level. This workout can be done progressively over the course of your training cycle. Start with 2 repeats and gradually progress to 6 repeats as you become fitter.

Time/Distance	Pace	Comments
10 Minutes	Easy Pace	Warm Up
1 Mile	RPE 14 - 15. Somewhat hard to hard pace. 10K race pace or 15 seconds per mile slower than 5K race pace	Your pace should feel hard but you should not be struggling.
1/4 Mile	Easy Pace	You can use 1/4 of active recovery or rest completely for 2 minutes.
1 Mile	RPE 14 - 15. Somewhat hard to hard pace. 10K race pace or 15 seconds per mile slower than 5K race pace	Keep repeating this pattern of 1 mile hard and 1/4 mile or 2 minutes of recovery for as many repeats as you desire. Start with just 2 repeats and gradually work up to 6 as you gain fitness.
1/4 Mile	Easy Pace	Recovery

Speed Endurance Ladder

Remember that a ladder is a workout in which you start with a specific run and work progressively up in distance or pace (up the ladder) or down in distance or pace (down the ladder). Here is a beginners speed endurance ladder. Unlike most ladder workouts, this one includes recovery periods. After a warm up, run 1/2 mile at RPE 14 to 15 (somewhat hard to hard) or current 10K pace, then recover with 1/4 mile at a comfortable pace. Increase your speed again to RPE 14 to 15 or 10K pace and run 3/4 mile. Recover with 1/4 mile at a comfortable pace and then return to RPE 14 to 15 or 10K pace for 1 mile. Finish with a cool down of 1/2 mile at an easy pace. You could reverse this workout by running "down the ladder" by starting with 1 mile followed by 3/4 mile and 1/2 mile. All of the runs being performed at RPE 14 to 15 or 10K pace with 1/4 mile of easy running in between to recover.

Time/Distance	Pace	Comments
10 Minutes	Easy Pace	Warm Up
1/2 Mile	RPE 14 to 15 or 10K race pace	This pace should be somewhat hard to hard
1/4 Mile	Comfortable Pace	Recovery
3/4 Mile	RPE 14 to 15 or 10K race pace	Keep running up the ladder
1/4 Mile	Comfortable Pace	Recovery
1 Mile	RPE 14 to 15 or 10K race pace	Top of the ladder
1/4 Mile	Easy Pace	Cool down

Speed Endurance Superset

A superset is a set of intervals that vary in both distance and pace. There are no recovery intervals in a superset. You switch between the various distances and speeds with no rest periods. This is a beginning level superset.

After a warm up, run 1/2 mile at RPE 14 to 15 or 10K race pace (somewhat hard to hard), then slow down to RPE 13 to 14 or about 10 seconds per mile slower than 10K pace for 3/4 mile followed by 1 mile RPE 12 to 13 or a somewhat hard pace. This should be about 20 seconds per mile slower than 10K race pace. This entire workout is preformed with no recovery intervals or rest.

Time/Distance	Pace	Comments
10 Minutes	Easy Pace	Warm Up
1/2 Mile	RPE 14 to 15 or 10K race pace	This pace should be somewhat hard to hard
3/4 Mile	RPE 13 to 14 or 10 seconds per mile slower than 10K pace	Slightly easier pace or somewhat hard
1 Mile	RPE 12 to 13 or 20 seconds per mile slower than your 10K race pace	Comfortable to somewhat hard
10 Minutes	Easy Pace	Cool Down

Strength Building Hill Workouts

Hill running is one the best and most efficient methods of improving your speed and performance. It improves your running specific strength, running economy, running mechanics, power, lactate turn point and aerobic conditioning. It also prepares you for the hills that you run into when you are racing.

There are three types of hill training that benefits runners.

•   Hills that are included as part of a longer training run.

•   Long hill repeats or one long consistent hill workout that is run at a strong, but maintainable pace.

•   Short hill repeats run at a fast pace.

Hill runs are not easy workouts. They should be run at a pace that feels fairly hard, but not so hard that you cannot complete the entire workout at your planned pace. How hard you run the hills depends upon your specific level of fitness.

Hill workouts are perfect for the treadmill. Many runners are located in areas that have few hills. Even if you are located in a hilly area, you will probably have problems finding hills that will work perfectly for your planned workout. The treadmill removes this problem by providing hills of any length and at a wide range of inclines. It allows you to structure hill work that is very specific to your goals and your level of fitness. Most treadmills will adjust from zero to 12 percent incline, which will work well for almost all of your hill workouts.

Hill Blasters

This is a standard hill workout that uses short runs up a moderate to steep grade. This training run is very good for building strength and power and well as boosting your lactate turn point.

Find a hill in your area that has a moderate to steep grade. If you don't have an appropriate hill in your area you can do this workout on a treadmill. Warm up for 10 to 15 minutes. If you are using a treadmill set the treadmill at 10 to 12 percent elevation, or the highest elevation available on your treadmill. Run for 1/10th of a mile at RPE 17 to 18. You should run at a pace that you can maintain for the entire workout, not just one repetition. You should not feel exhausted after one or two repetitions. If you are excessively fatigued, slow down your pace. After running uphill for 1/10th of a mile, jog back down the hill the hill or decrease the elevation of your treadmill to 1 percent and decrease your speed to an easy pace for one minute of recovery. Then run back up the hill at RPE 17 to 18 or increase the treadmill elevation back to 12 percent for another 1/10th of a mile before jogging back down for recovery.

Time/Distance	Pace	Comments
10 Minute	Easy Pace	Warm Up
1/10th Mile	Run uphill at RPE 17 - 18	If you are using a treadmill use 12% elevation
1/10th Mile	Easy recovery pace	Jog down the hill or decrease the treadmill elevation to 1%
1/10th Mile	Run uphill at RPE 17 - 18	Keep repeating this sequence for your desired number of repetitions.
1/10th Mile	Easy recovery pace	Start with 3 repetitions and increase the number gradually as your fitness increases

Hill Fartlek

Yes - I know - fartlek is a funny word, but it is actually a very common running term. It is a Swedish word that translates roughly as "speed play". Fartlek workouts are intended to be fun workouts. If there is such a thing as "fun" hill training, this is it.

This is an unstructured training run. The hard part of this run is finding an area that has rolling hills so that you are constantly changing elevation and terrain. If you don't have that type of terrain in your area you can do this on a treadmill. You decide when to throw in a hill and how steep to make the hill. You also decide what pace to run. Make this run different every time you perform it. When you do this run, do not plan your paces or elevations ahead of time. Just go with the flow and do whatever you feel like doing. The only rule is to change both pace and elevation frequently.

This is a good entry level hill workout for beginners. Have fun with this workout. The informal structure of this is something that you should enjoy and experiment with.

Time	Pace	Comments
10 Minutes	Warm Up	The added stress that hill running places on your muscles makes is especially important to warm up thoroughly
20 - 60 Minutes	Various paces between RPE 12 and 19	Various inclines between 1% and 12%

The Hill Climb

So far you have seen a short hill workout and a varied hill workout. Here is the final type of hill workout. A steady run up a long hill. This is a difficult workout that will challenge you both physically and mentally. If the shorter workouts are considered hill workouts, you may think of this one as a mountain workout. This workout will improve your strength, speed, power, lactate turn point and running economy. As with any hill workout, the problem is finding an appropriate hill. In this case you need a long one. If you cannot find a good hill or trail for this workout you will need to do it on the treadmill.

This workout is very simple. After your warm up run up a hill of moderate incline. If you are using a treadmill, set the elevation between 5% and 8%. Run up the hill at RPE 14 to 15. Run steadily for between 2 and 6 miles. Your exact amount of mileage will also depend upon your experience and fitness level. Use your own judgment. This workout should be difficult, but be careful not to over estimate your fitness level. It is better to start with less mileage and see how your body reacts than to injure yourself with excessive mileage. Remember that you will have to jog back down the hill unless you have transportation back to the bottom of the hill.

Time/Distance	Pace	Comments
10 Minutes	Easy Pace	Warm up thoroughly
2 to 6 miles	RPE 14 to 15	Run at a steady pace. Your pace should feel somewhat hard to hard. Remember that you have to run back down the hill.
10 Minutes	Easy Pace	Cool Down

Endurance Building Long Runs

Long runs are one of the key workouts to building endurance and are the cornerstone of long distance running. These long endurance runs are the workouts that, for many, bestow an identity to a distance runner. When the term "distance runner" comes up, it brings with it an image of a solitary athlete gliding smoothly along a rolling road or trail.

When many runners think of long runs they envision marathon running and training. Long runs are a key workout for marathon runners, but they are also used for all race distances and every level of runner including beginning runners. Long runs are the best way to build your endurance and also builds a base of fitness.

The long runs improve your endurance. They train your body to run for long distances without stopping. They strengthen your muscles, joints and tendons so that you can avoid injury and support our faster paced runs. Long runs also train your mind. Long runs toughen you mentally so that you develop the ability to keep going even though your body is screaming at you to stop. All of these improvements are essential if you are to perform to the best of your ability.

The training effects of long runs are cumulative. The payoff of these workouts build upon themselves week after week, month after month and year after year. You will get physically and mentally stronger. Your body will learn to store more and more energy providing glycogen, and your cardiovascular system will provide more and more oxygen to your muscles.

A long run should be included in your training program

from once a week to once every three weeks, depending upon your goal, your experience level and where you are in your training cycle. There are two different types of long runs:

•   **Easy Pace Long Runs** - When most runners think of long runs this is the workout that they are doing. The pace is between 30 seconds slower than marathon pace to over one minute slower than marathon pace. The distance is anywhere from 10 miles up to 30 miles or 1 hour to over 4 hours. The distance and time depends upon your goal race and your fitness level.

•   **Goal Pace Long Run** - This is a long run that is either partially or completely performed at your race goal pace. This long run can be used for any goal race distance, but is most commonly used for marathon training. If you are going to race a marathon, you must do some training at your goal race pace. The format can take several forms. It can be a long run in which a portion of it, usually the first part, is done at an easy pace and the last part is done at goal pace. This will train your body to run at goal pace for long distances while already fatigued. Goal pace can also be incorporated throughout a long run, much like a fartlek run. A fartlek run is a workout in which you change pace at your whim, without structure. In addition to multi pace runs, some medium distance long runs are done entirely at race pace.

Easy Paced Long Run

This is a basic endurance training long run. It is the same workout as the basic marathon training run that I refer to as "The Big Easy" in the marathon training schedule. The pace of this workout will vary from runner to runner, but should always be comfortable and "conversational" in nature or about RPE 12. You should be running easy enough that you can carry on a conversation but you should not be able to sing.

The distance of your first long run should be the distance of your longest run in the past three weeks. The distance of each subsequent long run should be increased by one or two miles depending upon the amount of time until your goal race and your fitness level. You should do a long run from one to three times per month. Once you reach 10 to 12 miles you should do these no more than every other week. These runs are performed at an easy pace, but should not be considered an easy run. The amount of time and distance involved make long runs a hard run and appropriate recovery time should be planned both before and after a long run.

Time/Distance	Pace	Comments
5 Minutes	Easy Pace	Warm Up
3 Miles to 23 Miles	RPE 12 to 13 - Comfortable Pace	Start with your longest run in the past 3 weeks. Add one or two miles to your long run each time. If you are training for a marathon you should extend your long run to 22 or 23 miles three weeks before your race.
5 Minutes	Easy Pace	Cool Down

Fast Finish Long Run

Long slow endurance running is a valuable training tool. But it does not prepare you to run at faster goal race pace. Fast finish long runs improve your running economy at race pace, mentally prepare you for the speed that you will be running in races and makes you more comfortable with your goal pace.

These workouts are performed by running at RPE 12 or a comfortable pace for the first portion of your long run and then speeding up to your goal pace for the last portion. If you are training for a marathon you finish at marathon pace. If your goal race is a 10K you finish at 10K pace.

For your first fast finish long run, do the last 1 mile at goal pace. For the ensuing runs, gradually increase the amount of goal pace running up to half of your entire long run. This workout should be done anywhere from once per month to once every two weeks.

Time/Distance	Pace	Comments
5 Minutes	Easy Pace	Warm Up
3 to 23 Miles	First Portion at RPE 12 to 13 - Comfortable pace followed by the second portion at goal pace	For your first workout do only the last mile at goal pace. In subsequent workouts gradually increase the distance of your goal pace portion until you are doing half of the workout at goal pace.
5 Minutes	Easy Pace	Warm Up

Long Run Fartlek

This is a long run with a little spice. Run your scheduled long run distance at a RPE 12 to 13 or a comfortable pace. Every two or three miles, increase your speed to anywhere between RPE 14 to 18 for between 400 meters and 1 mile. You choose what speed and how often you do these faster pace surges. There is no strict structure to this run. Do not use the same distance for all of your surges. Do some long surges and some short. This run should be fun, but also serves a valuable service. It prepares you for the different paces that you will be running during your races.

Time/Distance	Pace	Comments
5 Minutes	Easy Pace	Warm Up
3 to 23 Miles	RPE 12 - Comfortable pace with unstructured surges at between RPE 14 and 18.	This is a fun, unstructured run so throw in the surges whenever you feel like it. Have fun with this workout.
5 Minutes	Easy Pace	Cool Down

Go Farther and Get Faster Training Schedule

There are a nearly unlimited number of ways you could combine all of these speed and endurance workouts to go farther and get faster. It could be a simple as adding a longer run one every few weeks or as complex as a detailed weekly or biweekly schedule using all of these workouts. Any time you push yourself past your current limitations with a longer or faster run you are improving your running abilities. As a beginning runner you need to strike a balance between pushing yourself enough to improve but not so much that you get injured or burned out. In the following table, I have outlined a training schedule that is challenging enough to improve your performance but is still appropriate for your beginning level.

This is a 14 day schedule that includes one long run, one speed workout, one speed endurance run and one hill workout every seven days. Each of these workouts play a role in improving your speed, stamina, endurance and strength. Each time you repeat this cycle add more repeats or decrease your recovery time between repeats. You want to challenge yourself with each workout. Don't forget the rest and easy run days. You need sufficient rest to make sure your muscles get enough recovery time. I would also suggest rotating other workouts into your schedule. Don't always do the same speed workouts or the same hill workouts. Variety will keep you motivated and will challenge your body in different ways. If you do the same routine over and over again, your body "learns" the workouts and does not improve as much as it should. Changing workouts frequently will help avoid that.

Farther and Faster Training Schedule

Day	Workout	Comments
1	Run 2 miles at a comfortable pace	Run at your typical easy comfortable pace.
2	Lactate Turn point Cruiser - 20 Minutes	Keep your pace strong and steady at about RPE 14
3	Run 3 miles at a comfortable pace	You will alternate hard workouts with easy or rest days to insure sufficient recovery.
4	4 x 400 meter repeats	Run four repetitions of 400 meter repeats. These at RPE 18
5	Rest	Take the day off
6	Hill Blasters	Start with 3 repetitions. As you build your fitness level you should increase the number of repetitions.
7	Easy Pace Long Run	Start with the distance of your longest run in the past 3 weeks. You will build on that from here.
8	Rest	Take the day off to recovery from your long run effort.
9	3 x One Mile Repeats	Run 3 x One Mile Repeats. Keep your pace strong throughout your work repeats
10	Run 4 miles at a comfortable pace	These easy runs are always at around RPE 12
11	Beginners Ladder	Run 1 complete ladder
12	Rest	Take the day off
13	Hill Fartlek	Run for 30 minutes for your first attempt at this workout. You will add to this later
14	Long Run	A long run is scheduled for the last day of each week. Keep adding to the distance of your long run up to 12 miles. At that point start doing them only every other week.

Strengthening and Lengthening

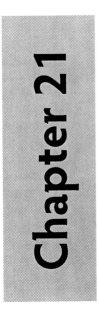

Strengthening and lengthening are two terms that go hand in hand. Strength training makes your muscles stronger and more powerful. It also improves your resistance to injuries. Lengthening or flexibility increases your range of motion, improves the elasticity of your muscles and also helps prevent injuries. Both are important in building up your running strength and overall fitness.

Do You Really Need Strength Training?

Is it absolutely necessary that you perform strength training as a runner? Not really - there are very few absolutes in this world. Will strength training help you avoid injuries? - You bet! Will it make you a better, more efficient runner? - No doubt about it! Will strength training improve your fitness level? - Of course! Will it help you lose and maintain your weight? - Yes, no question about it!

253

That being said there are many runners who never engage in strength training. In fact, there is a false impression out there that strength training will adversely affect your running. That false belief could not be further from the truth. Strength training isn't just for body builders and football players anymore. Runners of all levels, especially beginning runners, can and will benefit greatly from a properly designed strength-training program. In fact, most runners will never reach their peak level of performance without strength training. Running training programs in the past and still today have ignored the benefits of strength training. Many coaches and athletes have even avoided strength training because of the belief that any increase in muscle mass will slow down or decrease the endurance of the runner. Current research has proven that this is not true. Strength training is a vital component of any runners training regime.

As a beginning runner you may or may not have a base of muscular and connective tissue strength built up. If you are currently involved in strength training or participate in other sports that require strong, powerful muscles you already know the benefits of strength training. You also probably have a strong base of strength. If not, you would be well advised to add strength training into your exercise routine. Running is high intensity level activity. Running long distances or at a high intensity level without a strong base of strength is like building a house of cards. It can collapse when under stress because it does not have a strong foundation. If you do not have a strong base and core your body can react in the same way. You won't completely collapse but you can suffer from a long list of running related injuries that are related to your lack of a strong core and base of running strength.

In addition to the fitness, health and weight loss benefits, there are many other positive aspects of strength training. The most important benefits to a beginning runner are injury prevention and running economy.

Injury Prevention

The repetitive stresses of running places a lot of demands upon your muscles, ligaments, tendons and joints. As a new runner your muscles are probably not used to that much activity and they may rise up in protest. They are saying "what the heck is this person doing to us? We've never had to do this before"! Your abused muscles and tendons voice their complaints in the form of soreness or injury. Nothing will totally prevent the occurrence of injuries. However, strength training will provide a defense against overuse injures. It is like your muscles calling in some reinforcements. You are telling your muscles and tendons that you need them to grow stronger to support your new activity. They respond by increasing in strength and size. When injuries do occur, your improved level of strength will decrease both the severity of the injury and your recovery time.

Strength training protects your body from injuries in several ways. Your muscles fibers themselves are strengthened which will help prevent muscle pulls and tears. Muscle mass is increased which will help provide support to your joints, which are absorbing much of the impact of running. All of your connective tissues, which include ligaments and tendons, are made stronger. This will help you avoid strains, sprains and tendonitis.

Running Economy

You may have heard the term "economy of motion". That term refers to the ability to create and maintain movement or motion using the least amount of energy possible. Running economy is very similar. It is a measure of how economical you are at running or how "easy" you are running. When you run you want to move easily, smoothly and fluidly, using the least amount of energy possible. Running economy is improved by maximizing stride length, maintaining stride rate, improving running form and running smoothly and effortlessly. Strength training provides the base for all of these improvements. Nearly all of the runners that I coach tell me that their running feels smoother and they feel that they are running with less effort after a period of general and running specific strength training.

Beginning Strength Training for Runners

The following exercises are basic beginning level strength training exercises that are great for improving both your overall strength and your running specific strength. Try to perform these exercises two times per week. I would suggest doing your strength workouts after your run rather than before. If you perform strength training before you run your muscles will already be fatigued and your running workout will be more difficult and of lower quality.

Most of the strength training exercises I will be recommending are body weight exercises. You can perform these exercises in your home, at the track, in the park or even your office. Many exercise books include strength exercises that require the use of expensive equipment or a gym membership. Of course, you can do these exercises in a gym or you could purchase additional strength training equipment for your home. But at the beginning level there is no need to do that. My goal for you as a beginning runner is to make strength training easy and convenient. You do not need that special equipment or expensive fitness club memberships. All you need is your running shoes, small hand weights, a willingness to do the exercises and a few extra minutes at the end of your daily running workout.

Later in your running life as your progress to higher levels of fitness and performance it will become beneficial to use some specialized exercise equipment. But for now it is not necessary. Keeping things easy and convenient will help you make running a lifetime activity.

Push Ups

This is a basic strength exercise that will strengthen the muscles of your upper chest, shoulders and triceps.

• Begin face down on the floor supporting yourself with your hands approximately shoulder width apart and your arms extended. Your feet can be together or up to 12 inches apart. Keep your body in a straight, neutral position. Do not arch your back. Contract your abdominal muscles to stabilize your trunk and spine.

• Slowly lower your body until your chest touches the floor. Push off the floor and return to the starting position. Repeat until you are fatigued.

• Breath throughout the exercise. Exhale on the upward portions and inhale on the downward portion.

• If this exercise is too difficult start with modified knee push ups in which you support your lower body on your knees instead of your feet. As your strength increases you will be able to graduate to standard push ups.

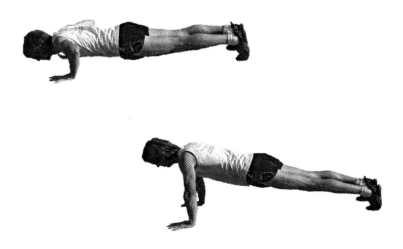

Biceps Curl

This exercise will build the strength of your biceps muscle on the front of your upper arm. The biceps muscle is difficult to strengthen without the use of some simple equipment. You can use hand weights, resistance tubing or you could even improvise using canned goods or buckets of water. Do one or two sets of 15 to 20 repetitions.

•   Standing upright, grasp the weight with your palms facing away from the front of your body. Contract your abdominal muscles to stabilize your trunk and spine. Keep your upper arms against your ribs and perpendicular to the floor.

•   Slowly raise the weight by flexing your arms at your elbows. Keep your upper arms stationary. Raise the weight to the limit of your natural motion. Slowly return to the starting position.

•   Breath throughout the exercise. Exhale on the upward portions and inhale on the downward portion. Do not arch your back. Keep your body still and straight. Control the weight throughout the exercise.

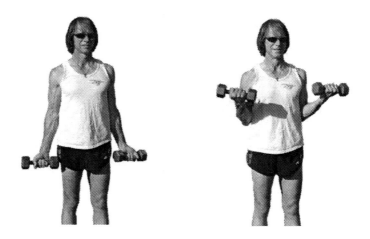

Bench Dips

This exercise will develop your triceps muscle which is located on the back of your upper arm. All you need to perform this exercise is a bench or a high step. You can also do this exercise on the bleachers at your local school track.

•   Sit on the bench or step with your palms down and gripping the edge of the bench. Slide your feet out in front of you so that you are supporting yourself on your heels and hands.

•   Slowly lower yourself until your elbows are bent to approximately 90 degrees. Keeping your elbows pointing behind you push yourself back up by straightening your arms. Repeat this until you are fatigued. Breath throughout the exercise. Exhale on the upward portions and inhale on the downward portion.

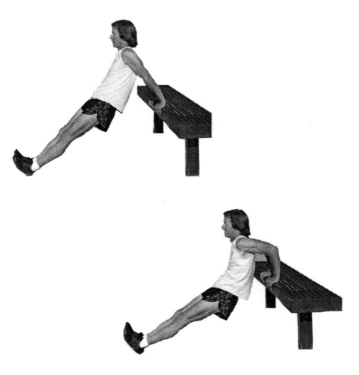

Bent Over Row

This exercise works the muscles of your upper back. Just as your biceps, this muscle is difficult to work without some simple equipment. You can use hand weights or resistance tubing to perform this workout. Do one or two sets of 15 to 20 repetitions.

•   Support yourself on a bench with one knee and one arm. Your back should be straight and parallel to the floor. Contract your abdominal muscles to stabilize your trunk

•   Grasp the weight with your hand in a neutral position like your are holding a candle or a glass of water. Your arm should be fully extended, with the weight on the floor. Slowly pull the weight straight up until it is approximately chest level. Keep your elbow close to your body. Slowly extend your arm and allow the weight to return to the floor. Control the weight all the way down.

•   Concentrate on pulling with the latissimus dorsi muscles of your back. You should feel as if you are contracting your shoulder blade.

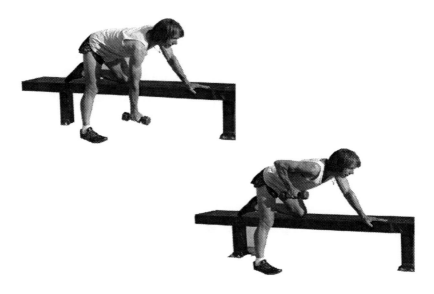

Core Stabilization

Strong core muscles are essential for proper running technique and endurance. Hold each exercise for 20 to 30 seconds. Perform 1 set.

• Lie face down on a mat or on a soft grassy area. Support your weight with your feet and forearms. Tuck your pelvis so that your hips are pressed forward and your body is straight. Hold this position for 20 to 30 seconds.

• Now lift your left arm and hold it straight out so that it is above your head. Hold for 20 to 30 seconds. Return the left arm to the support position and lift your right arm above your head and hold for 20 to 30 seconds. Return the right arm to the support position and lift your left foot off of the mat and hold for 20 to 30 seconds. Return the left foot to the mat and lift the right foot and hold for 20 to 30 seconds.

• Here comes the fun part. Lift your right arm and left foot at the same time. You should now be supporting your body with your left forearm and your right foot. Hold for 20 to 30 seconds. Now return the right arm and left foot to the mat and lift your left arm and right foot. Hold for 20 to 30 seconds.

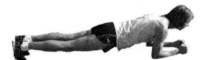

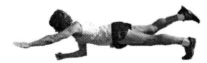

Squats

This is a body weight exercise that will strengthen the muscles on the front and back of your thigh. Perform one set of 20 repetitions.

•   Stand in an upright position with your feet shoulder width apart. Hold your chest up and out. Pinch your shoulder blades together. Keep your head up. Contract your abdominal to stabilize your trunk.

•   Slowly lower your body by allowing your knees and hips to flex. Maintain an erect body position. Lower your body until your thighs are nearly parallel to the floor. Do not allow your knees to move in front of your toes. As you lower your body raise your arms in front of you.

•   Slowly raise your body back up to the starting position by extending your knees and hips. Breath throughout the exercise. Exhale on the upward portions and inhale on the downward portion. Do not arch your back.

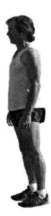 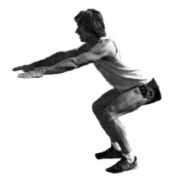

Calf Raise

This is another basic body weight exercise that will strengthen your calf muscles and will also condition your Achilles tendon. Perform one set of 20 repetitions on each leg.

•   Stand with one foot on a bench or step. Your toes and the ball of your foot should be on the step with your heel hanging off the edge. Hold your other foot up and behind you.

•   Extend your foot so that your heel is raised up and your foot is on its toes. Slowly lower your heel until it is slightly below the step and you feel a slight stretch in your calf muscle. Repeat for your desired number of repetitions. Repeat this exercise with the other foot. Breath throughout the exercise. Exhale on the upward portions and inhale on the downward portion.

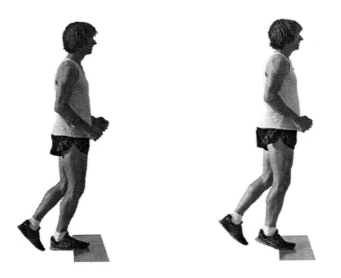

Bench Step Ups

This is a body weight exercise that is specifically designed to improve your running strength, running economy and running form. Perform 1 set of 20 repetitions on each leg.

•   Stand directly in front of a step bench that is 18 to 24 inches high. Place one foot (support foot) flat on the bench. With most of your weight on the heel of your support foot, forcefully push off with the support leg. A the same time drive your other knee up as in a running motion.

•   Slowly lower your driving leg back to the ground in the original starting position. Repeat for the desired number of repetitions.

•   Repeat this exercise using the other leg as the support leg. Breath throughout the exercise. Inhale on the downward portions and exhale on the upward portion. Keep your back in a vertical position. Do not allow the knee of the support leg to extend in front of the foot.

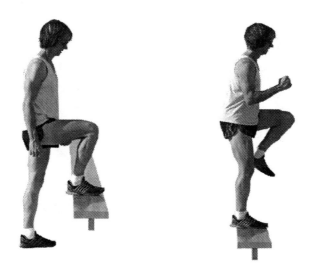

One-Leg Bench Squats

This is a body weight exercise that is excellent for developing running specific strength because it is performed in a running position. Do 1 set of 20 repetitions on each leg.

•   Contract your abdominal muscles to stabilize your trunk and spine. Place one foot (rear foot) behind you on a bench that is 6 to 12 inches high. Your other foot (forward foot) should be flat on the floor and directly under you. Bend your forward knee until it is at approximately a 90-degree angle. Do not let your knee extend in front of your foot. Slowly straighten your forward leg and return to the starting position. Repeat this exercise using the other leg as the lead leg.

•   Breath throughout the exercise. Inhale on the downward portions and exhale on the upward portion. Keep your back in a vertical position. Do not allow the knee of the forward leg to extend in front of the foot.

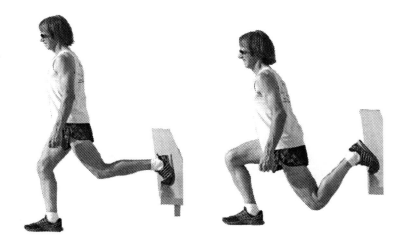

Lunge

This exercise is one of my favorites for building running specific strength. It is basically an exaggerated walking stride. The running specific motions of this exercise will give you a good muscle burn.

- Stand in an upright position. Contract your abdominal muscles to stabilize your trunk and spine. Take a long step forward with one leg. Keep the knee and foot of the forward leg aligned. Slowly flex the forward knee until the thigh is parallel to the floor. At the same time lower the knee of the trailing leg toward the floor. Do not allow the knee of the forward leg to extend in front of the foot. The knee of the rear leg should stop approximately 2 inches above the floor. Keep your upper body in a vertical position. Forcefully push off with the forward leg and bring it back into position with the trailing leg. You should now be back in the starting position.

- Repeat this exercise using the other leg as the forward leg. Keep your back in a vertical position. Do not allow the knee of the forward leg to extend in front of the foot. Do not lock your knees at any time during this exercise.

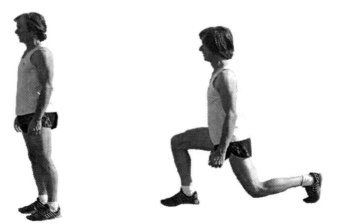

Stretching for Beginning Runners

In the chapter on Aches and Pains I outlined the 5 primary types of stretching and which ones are most appropriate for you as a beginning runner. The five stretching methods are static stretching, passive stretching, dynamic stretching or drills, ballistic stretching, proprioceptive neuromuscular facilitation (PNF) and active isolated (AI) stretching. As I discussed in that chapter, studies have shown that the safest and most effective methods are dynamic drills before your workout and static or AI stretching after your run.

In recent years there has been a lot of controversy concerning the effectiveness of stretching in preventing injuries and enhancing performance. In the past it was an accepted fact that all athletes should perform stretching exercises both before and after any physical activity. At that time it was thought that stretching your muscles before a run would lengthen the muscle so that it would be less likely to suffer from a strain or tear when it is placed under the high stresses of running.

More recent and detailed studies are showing that static stretching before an activity may not help prevent injuries and may in fact contribute to injuries and decrease your performance. An investigation at the University of Minnesota[1] concluded that increasing your range of motion beyond your normal functional level is not beneficial and could cause injury and decrease performance levels.

That is just one of many scientific studies that agree that the best way to decrease injury and improve performance is by doing dynamic flexibility exercises before you run rather than the common static stretches. Gentle static stretching should still be done after you run to maintain your range of motion.

---

1   Minn Med. 2003 May;86(5):58-61

Dynamic Warm Up Flexibility Drills

Dynamic warm up drills are active functional exercises in which you move your limbs through their full, natural and functional range of motion. You are not forcing your range of motions outside of what is required to perform your chosen sport of running. These are beginning level dynamic drills. Always warm up with 3 to 5 minutes of brisk walking or easy running before you do these exercises. A warm up is necessary to increase the flow of blood to your muscles, lubricate your joints and raise your body temperature.

This type of stretching uses the momentum generated during the dynamic motion to propel your muscle into a slightly extended range of motion but not past your functional range. That makes this type of stretch very safe and effective at preparing your muscles for the activity that follows. Dynamic warm up drills help develop your speed, power and neuro-muscular coordination as well as providing flexibility.

Dynamic exercises should always be done before your actual running workout. You should follow your run or workout with a series of gentle static stretches.

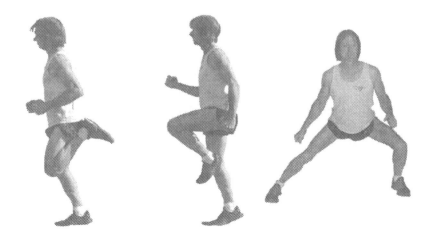

Walking Lunge

Take a long, exaggerated step forward with one leg. Drive your knee high and reach out as far as possible. Slowly flex your forward knee until your thigh is parallel to the ground. At the same time lower the knee of your trailing leg toward the ground. Do not allow the knee of your forward leg to extend in front of your foot. The knee of your trailing leg should stop approximately 2 inches above the ground, not touch the ground. Your upper body should remain in a vertical position.

Forcefully push off with our forward leg, keeping most of your weight over your forward heel. At the same time cycle your trailing leg through and perform the same motion as described above. Keep performing these cycling motions so that you are moving forward with a walking lunge. Keep going for about 20 meters.

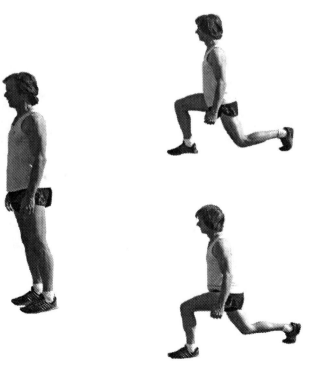

Walking High Knees Drill

Using a short stride and bouncing on your toes, take a step with an exaggerated high stride. Drive your knee as high as possible on each stride. As you drive your knee high bounce up on the toes of your opposite foot.

Keep cycling your legs through this motion so that you are moving slowly forward over the ground with the exaggerated high knee motion and bouncing on your opposite foot. Keep going for about 20 meters.

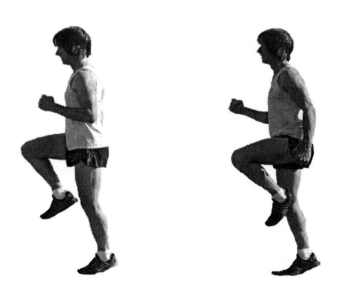

Heel Kick Drill

Begin by performing a slow jog. Using a short stride and bouncing on your toes, raise your heels as high as possible behind your body. Attempt to bounce your heels off your buttocks. Most of the movement should be with your lower leg. Concentrate on raising your heels as high as possible and staying on the balls of your feet with a bouncing motion. Keep moving forward for about 20 meters.

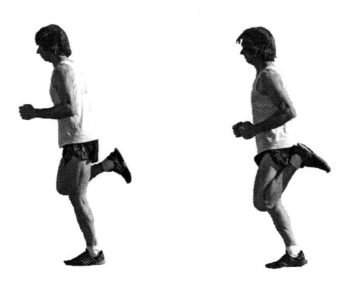

Walking Side Lunge Drill

This drill is similar to the walking lunge exercise except you will be moving to the side instead of forward. Take a long, exaggerated step sideways with one leg. Slowly flex your lunging knee until your thigh is parallel to the ground. At the same time your trailing leg should remain straight and close to the ground. Your upper body should remain in a vertical position.

Forcefully push off with your lunging leg, keeping most of your weight over your forward heel. Stand upright and bring your feet back together. Keep performing these motions so that you are moving sideways. Keep going for about 20 meters, then repeat going the opposite direction.

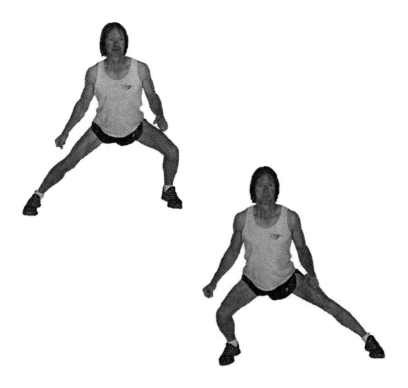

Arm Swing Drill

Standing in a relaxed upright position. Holding your arms out to the side swing them forward so that they cross in front of your body. Now swing them back through your natural and functional range of motion. Keep doing this for about 30 seconds.

Now hold your arms at your side in a running position with your elbows flexed to about 90%. Keep your shoulders relaxed. Swing your arms forward and back in an exaggerated running motion. Keep going for about 30 seconds.

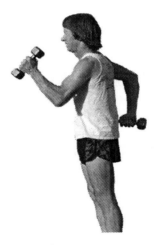

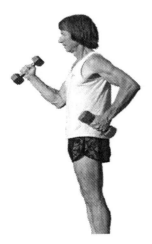

Static Cool Down Stretches

Static stretches are the most commonly performed stretches. When doing these stretches you assume the specific stretch position and hold it for about 20 to 30 seconds. You should stretch only until you feel a slight pull on your muscle. Never stretch to the point of pain and never bounce or make rapid movements. Do these stretches after your training run or race, not before.

These stretches will increase the flexibility of the "belly" or main part of your muscles as well as decreasing the sensitivity of tension receptors in your muscle. When the sensitivity of these receptors are lessened it allows your muscle to relax and lengthen even further.

Some people use the terms static stretching and passive stretching interchangeably. They are not the same. Static and passive stretches are the same. The difference is in how they are performed. You provide the force required for static stretching by using an opposing muscle group, using your body weight or pushing and pulling. When doing passive stretching you relax completely and let a machine or a helper provide the stretching force.

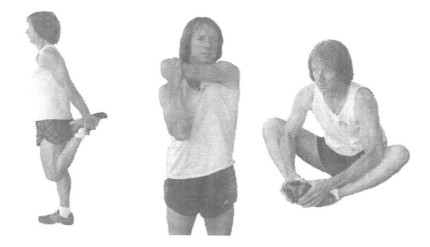

Hamstring Stretch

Lie on your back in a supine position. Keep your right foot on the ground with your knee bent at 90 degrees. Raise your left leg up, grab it below your ankle and pull it toward your shoulders. Pull your leg until your feel a slight pull. Hold that position for about 20 seconds. Switch your leg positions and repeat.

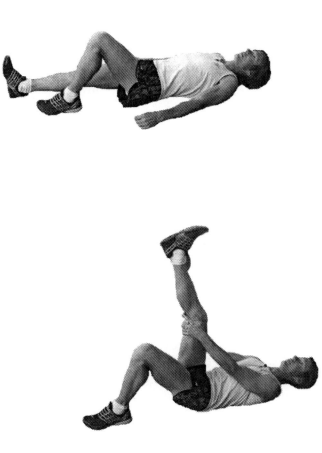

Hip Stretch

This exercise will stretch the iliopsoas muscle on the front of your hip. Move your right leg forward until your knee is directly over your ankle. Your left leg should be stretched out behind you with your knee on the ground. Now lower and push your hips down and forward to create a gentle stretch. Hold this position for 20 to 30 seconds. Switch your leg positions and repeat.

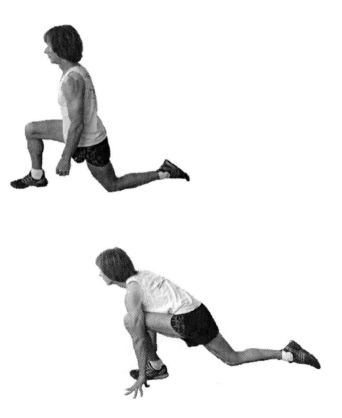

Quadriceps Stretch

While standing on your left foot, pull your right foot up toward your right hip. Keep your lower leg aligned with your thigh. Do not pull your lower leg to the right or left. Pull until you feel a gentle stretch. Hold this position for 20 to 30 seconds. Switch leg positions and repeat.

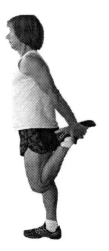

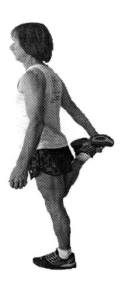

Butterfly Stretch

This is an exercise that will stretch the adductor (groin) muscles of your inner thigh. Start in a sitting position with your knees out and the soles of your feet together. Grab your toes and pull them gently upward. At the same use your elbows to gently push outward on your knees. You should feel a slight stretch on your inner thigh. Hold this position for about 20 to 30 seconds.

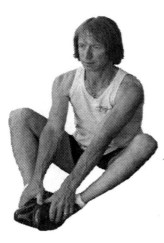

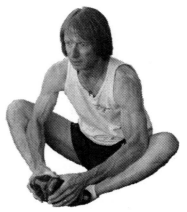

Pretzel Stretch

This exercise will stretch your upper back, lower back, hips and illiotibial band. Start is a sitting position with your right leg straight. Bend your left knee and cross it over your right leg so that it rests on the outside of your right knee. Now place your right elbow on the outside of your left knee. While supporting your body with your left hand twist your body to the left. Turn and look in that same direction. Hold that position for 20 to 30 seconds. Switch leg positions and repeat.

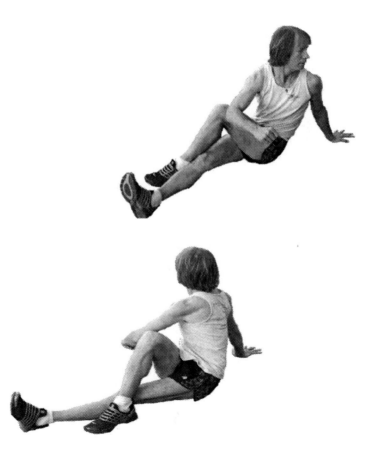

Calf Stretch

There are two muscles in your calf that you should stretch. The largest and most visible muscle is called the gastrocnemius muscle. This is the large one you can see on the back of your lower leg. Underneath your gastrocnemius muscle is your soleus muscle. Your gastrocnemius muscle does most of the work when your knee is straight. When your knee is bent your soleus muscle contributes more work.

To stretch your gastrocnemius muscle lie face down with your arms supporting your upper body in a push up position. Place your left foot over the back of your right ankle. Keep your right leg straight. With your toes flat on the ground push back so that your right heel is forced towards the ground. Hold that position for 20 to 30 seconds. Reverse leg positions and repeat.

To stretch your soleus muscle perform the same exercise except bend your leg at the knee. This will bring your soleus muscle more into the stretch.

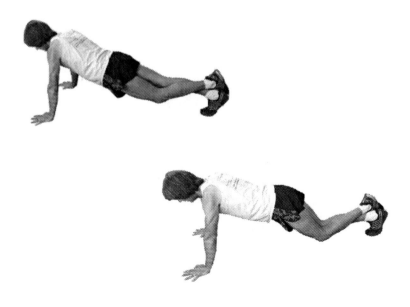

Shoulder Stretch

This exercise will stretch your shoulder, triceps and upper back. Grab your left elbow with your right hand and pull it gently across your chest toward your left shoulder. Hold that position for about 20 to 30 seconds. Reverse your arm positions and repeat.

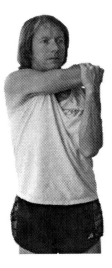

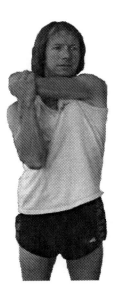

Treadmill Training

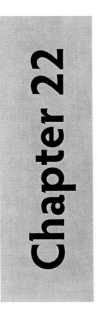

In the not too distant past, the term treadmill brought up all sorts of negative images. The definition of "treadmill" is - "A habitual, laborious, often tiresome course of action." That is enough to give a runner a textbook case of the "willies!." The only runners seen on treadmills in those days, were hooked up to hoses, plugs and wires to provide researchers with information on respiration, VO_2 max and stresses on joints and muscles. That image will scare away even the most dedicated runners.

Treadmills of the past did their part to earn their reputation as an instrument of torture. They were big, clunky, ugly and loud enough to drown out a jet engine at full throttle. They were hard to look at and hard to run on. The belts did not operate smoothly and the whole machine rocked and rolled like the deck of a sailboat in a squall.

On top of all this, treadmills were stigmatized. Runners simply did not believe that running on a treadmill, was "real" running. They also thought that anyone caught running on one, was not a "real" runner. Even if you wanted to run on the treadmill, you wouldn't risk the humiliation of being seen on it.

In those days, runners did not trust the training benefits of treadmill training. They felt that the treadmill would not give them the same physiological improvements that free range running did.

Well - things have changed. Beginning in the early 1990's, the treadmill boom began. In 1987, 4.4 million Americans owned and exercised on treadmills. Ten years later, in 1997, 36.1 million owned treadmills -a whopping 772% increase. One would assume that an increase of that magnitude would be due to an increase in the number of runners. But that was not the case. According to the Fitness Products Council and American Sports Data, Inc., the number of Americans that participated in running as a fitness activity actually decreased from 32.9 million in 1987 to 32.3 million in 1997. So, the increase must have been due to an incredible change in the attitude of runners towards treadmills.

In 2002 a record 43.4 million runners did at least part of their training on a treadmill. That trend is continuing. Just look around your neighborhood gym. What is the most popular machine? In most cases it is the treadmills. Treadmills are not just for beginning runners. Even top level competitive runners do some training on the treadmill.

This growth in the popularity of treadmills did not stop in 1997. In 2002, a record 43.4 million runners did at least a portion of their training runs on the treadmill. While not matching the exponential growth of the 1990's, that is still a lofty 17% increase.

So, what is driving this recent surge in treadmill popularity? Could it be that runners of today are a bit less elitist? That is probably, at least partly, true. The current crop of runners is a much more diverse group. They come from many different backgrounds, have many different goals and run for many different reasons. Some are highly fit and some are not so fit. Some are world class athletes while others are just learning to run.

This diversification has been very good for the sport of running. It has made what was once a sport with low participation numbers into one of the most popular forms of exercise and competition.

The sporting goods industry took note of this and started to design treadmills that were far more user friendly. The loud and ugly machines of the past were replaced with sleek, quiet and easy to use pieces of exercise equipment. The manufacturers also added more runner friendly features, such as programmed workouts, calorie counters, elevation, and displays that made the treadmill workouts more interactive, interesting and less boring. They made the treadmills more durable, more accessible and easier to maintain.

The treadmill made it easier for a beginning runner to stick to their training program. If it was cold or dark, they could just hop on the treadmill. It took away an excuse for not running. This made the treadmill a very popular item for new runners, fitness enthusiasts and those trying to lose weight.

It was not just beginners or dieters that began to use the treadmill frequently. Experienced runners and even elite competitive runners started to incorporate treadmill runs into their training program.

I first started to run on the treadmill in the 1980's. It all started on a cold, winter day. Rather than run outside in the cold and on the ice, I ran on a treadmill at the gym. I expected to hate the treadmill workout and dreaded even starting. Then, a funny thing happened. I actually enjoyed the run! There was a television in the gym, in front of the treadmill. It gave me a chance to get in some guilt-free television time. I was warm, comfortable and had easy access to water.

Not only was it more comfortable, but the workout was of a higher quality than I would have gotten had I tried to run on the snow and ice. I was able to concentrate on form and pace rather than focusing on my footing on the slick roads.

Shortly after that training run, I purchased my first treadmill. I started to do nearly all of my "bad weather" workouts on the treadmill. At first, I defined "bad weather" as blizzard conditions. That definition soon changed. The more time I spent on the treadmill, the more I liked it and the more broad my definition of bad weather became. "Bad weather" had now become anytime the temperature was below 50 degrees. I live in Colorado, so that is half the year.

I had now become a treadmill "junkie" and I was not alone. Many top runners, including elite world class runners, now do at least some of their workouts on a treadmill.

Dr. Christine Clark is a physician and marathon runner who lives in Alaska. With two young children to care for and frigid temperatures to contend with, she turned to the treadmill for training. She did nearly all of her training on the treadmill. So, how did she do, training on the treadmill? Well, she qualified for the marathon in the Sydney Olympics with a time of 2:33:31 in the Olympic trials at Columbia, South Carolina. Not Bad!

Norwegian marathon runner, Ingrid Kristiansen, set a world record of 2:21:06 at the London Marathon in 1985. Where did she do most of her workouts during the cold Norwegian winter? You guessed it. On the treadmill.

So, I no longer hide my treadmill. I readily admit that I do a large portion of my workouts on the treadmill. I incorporate treadmill workouts into my training plan. Why? Because treadmills are for "real" runners and the benefits of treadmill running are for real.

Treadmill Pros and Cons

As a running coach and a personal trainer, I get questions concerning the advantages and disadvantages of treadmill training from all types of clients. My running clients are concerned about the training effects of running on the treadmill. My personal training clients that are more interested in overall fitness and my weight loss clients, have questions concerning calorie burn and health benefits.

For fitness, health and weight loss purposes, there are really no disadvantages to treadmill training. A calorie burned on a treadmill is the same as a calorie burned during any other activity. Cardiovascular fitness is improved at a similar rate whether you run on a treadmill or outside on the road or track. The treadmill provides many added benefits for this type of user, including injury prevention, safety, convenience and improved exercise adherence. The treadmill also provides these same benefits to competitive runners. Fitness gained from running on the treadmill have been shown to be very similar to training effects from free range running. In some cases, treadmill training provides even greater training benefits. An example of this is the consistent pace of the treadmill. Many training programs require workouts that are performed at a precise pace and distance. The treadmill makes maintaining an exact pace and judging the precise distance much easier.

There are some disadvantages for runners. These disadvantages are related to the lack of specificity when training for road or track racing. There is a rule of training called the rule of specificity" that says training should closely mimic the activity you are training for. There are very definite differences between treadmill running and free range running that violate this rule.

Pros

Adverse Weather

You look out your living room window. The wind is howling, the mercury in your thermometer is shivering at the bottom of the scale and the snow is piling up on your driveway. You have a five mile tempo run planned. Are you going to lace 'em up and head out? Unless you are about 400 meters short of a full mile, you are going to stay huddled in front of your fireplace!

It situations like that, a treadmill is the perfect answer. You can perform any of your training runs in the safety and comfort of your own home or at your gym.

Poor weather conditions are the bane of a distance runner's existence. There are a few die hard's out there that still enjoy running in the rain, snow and cold, but most runners, including myself, do not like it. A treadmill takes the weather factor out of the equation. You can always hop on your treadmill and do nearly any workout that you could have done outdoors. If ice or snow is present, running on the treadmill will certainly provide a better workout than running outside in those conditions. If you are running outside on ice or snow, you must be very cautious of your footing. It is nearly impossible to concentrate on your form or pacing when running on ice. It is also very difficult to maintain your planned pace, since you must slow down on such a slippery surface. The bulky or multi-layer clothing that you must wear in cold weather can disturb your stride and arm action.

High wind can also create havoc with your workout. Most competitive runners have a specific pace or intensity level planned for each workout. If you are running into a head wind, your pace will drop in relation to the intensity of the workout. And visa versa, if you have a tail wind your pace will be higher in relation to your intended run.

Cold weather alone will probably not adversely affect your run. But, for some runners, cold weather becomes an excuse not to do their planned workout. This is especially a problem for beginning runners. A treadmill removes all excuses for not running. Cold weather can also cause some breathing problems for runners with asthma. Running in a warm, climate controlled environment can help alleviate these problems. Safety is also an issue in some weather conditions. A slip on the ice or snow can cause serious injury that could put a quick halt to your racing and training season.

Cold, ice and snow are not the only weather related problems a runner must deal with. Hot weather can create an even more serious situation. Dehydration, heat exhaustion and heat stroke are very serious conditions that are frequently encountered by runners. Each of these conditions are caused by a combination of high heat and insufficient fluids. Running on a treadmill in a climate controlled environment with fluids readily available will take away all chances of developing these problems.

Speed Work/Interval Training

As a beginning runner, you will not be doing a lot of speed work. But later on when you want to improve your speed and level of fitness you will be doing a lot of speed work and interval training. Successful interval training depends upon running the repeats at a fairly precise speed and at a precise distance. It is hard for most runners to accurately judge pace while training at the track and becomes even more difficult when training on the open road. When training on the track, you at least know the exact distance you are running, but on the open road, it is all guesswork. There are some fairly accurate GPS training watches available that use satellite information to give you your pace and distance. These have proven to be fairly accurate, but are still not as precise as treadmill running.

The primary goal of running training is to improve your fitness and endurance. To do that you must consistently challenge yourself. It is very easy to subconsciously slow down when you begin to fatigue. The treadmill will not let you do that. It will keep you at your training pace for the duration of your workout unless you purposely slow down the machine

When doing interval training on a treadmill, you can set the pace and be assured that you are running at that speed throughout the repeat. The treadmill does not allow you to slow down or speed up. It forces you to maintain your target pace throughout the repeat or workout.

Consistent Pacing

When you begin to fatigue during your outside training runs, you may sub-consciously slow down. You do not realize that you are slowing down because you feel like you are running at the same rate of perceived exertion. In other words, you still believe that you are running at your goal pace. The accumulating effects of fatigue makes your goal pace feel harder and harder, so you slow down in response. This unintentional reduction in your pace can have a negative affect on the quality of your workout. This problem with inconsistent pace can happen in all workouts from speed work to long runs.

The treadmill will force you to maintain the pace that you had planned for the workout. The only way to slow down is to intentionally reduce the speed of the treadmill. This consistent pacing benefit can actually make treadmill training a higher quality workout than track or road training.

Easy Runs

Many runners, even beginners, like to run fast. But you cannot run hard and fast all of the time. Your muscles need time to rest and recover. Without that recovery time, you will not be able to complete your harder workouts at an optimal pace and quality.

Running easy is hard. In fact, running easy is one of the hardest things to do for many runners. Easy runs are necessary to allow your muscles to recover from hard, intense or long running sessions, but it can be very difficult to run at a pace easy enough to allow for muscle recovery. It can feel very slow and therefore many runners have a tendency to perform their easy runs at too fast a pace.

The treadmill fixes this problem. Once you determine your easy pace, it is a simple matter to set the treadmill at that pace and jump on. As long as you don't give into temptation and increase the speed of the machine, you will stay at your easy pace for the duration of the session. Maintaining an easy pace on your rest days will allow your muscles to stay fresh and will improve the quality of your harder training runs and avoid overtraining problems.

Beginning runners can also benefit by using the treadmill for easy runs. It is important for a new runner to strengthen unused tendons and muscles gradually before doing any intense or fast training. Setting the treadmill at an easy pace will help avoid any tendency to run faster than they should.

Hill Training

Hill running is one of the best and most efficient workouts for building running strength, running economy and improving race performance. The problem is that many runners live in areas that have few hills, if any. So, what do you do if you live in a hill challenged area? Simple - get on your treadmill. Most treadmills will elevate from 1 percent to 12 percent. Some elevate as high as 15%. There are some newer models that also decline 2 or 3 percent, which would be great training for races with some downhill sections, such as the Boston Marathon or trail races.

The elevation selections will allow you to closely mimic nearly any outside trail or road race. Even if you have access to hills in your area, the nearly unlimited variety of possible hill workouts on your treadmill will give you a greater variety of hill training options.

The treadmill not only supplies hills to those without hills, it also removes hills for those that don't want them. Many runners that live in mountain communities have problems finding a route that does not have hills. There are many times, especially during easy runs and periods of rest and recovery, that you do not want to run on hills. The treadmill will flatten the most hilly terrain!

Long Runs

You will not be doing long runs during this beginners program. But as you progress to higher and higher levels of fitness you will begin to do a weekly or biweekly long run. To most runners, the term long run brings up visions of running long distances in parks, on roads or urban trails. There are many great benefits of doing long runs on that type of terrain. However, more and more runners are doing at least some of their long runs on the treadmill. Many do all of their winter long runs on the treadmill to avoid weather related problems.

Running long on a treadmill sounds boring. But for that matter, so is running outside for long periods of time. When doing long runs on the treadmill you can watch television or listen to music to help alleviate boredom. I like to tape marathons or other running events and watch them while I run. I also enjoy watching running movies. Any movie will entertain you while you run, but I find that running movies keep me motivated.

The quality of your long runs can also be improved by running on the treadmill. The precise pace control will allow you to keep the pace down when necessary. It will keep you from running too fast during the first part of your long run. It will also keep you at a quality pace if you are doing goal pace long runs. It can be very difficult to maintain that quality goal pace in the later stages of your long run. The treadmill will keep you at that goal pace and you don't even have to think about it. This is essential for marathon training if you decide to set a goal of completing a marathon. During the last 6 to 8 miles of a marathon, it becomes very difficult to maintain your pace. In order to run your best marathon, you must practice maintaining your goal pace when you are very fatigued. Since the treadmill does not get tired, you must push the button to slow it down. So, the machine will keep you on your pace unless you make the decision to reduce your speed.

When doing your long runs on a treadmill, you are also near all of your water and fluid replacement drinks. No need to hide fluids in a bush or carry them with you. You are also just steps from a bathroom. No more quick trips behind the bushes.

Injury Prevention/Rehabilitation

Running on concrete and asphalt day in and day out places a lot of stress on the connective tissues in your legs. This can lead to potential overuse injuries.

High quality treadmills that are produced today give you a stable, but more forgiving surface. Treadmills are available in a fairly wide range of surface "softness". The firmness of the treadmill is determined by a combination of the running deck and the suspension system. Some are designed to more closely mimic the firm asphalt or concrete surface of the road and others are designed with a lot of "give" in order to provide a very soft ride for heavy runners or those with injury problems. There are even some machines available that are adjustable to different levels of shock absorption.

Programmed Workouts

Most quality treadmills have pre-programmed workouts that are designed for anything from weight loss to 10K races. This feature makes it easy for runners that are not interested in designing their own program.

For those that do develop their own training programs, many treadmills have the ability to store custom workouts. You just manually adjust the treadmill as you run. The treadmill will "remember" the workout. The next time you do that workout, the treadmill makes all of the adjustments automatically. Some of the newer, high tech treadmills even have the ability to download custom workouts over the internet.

Mental Toughness

The sport of running is a solitary activity that requires self-motivation, discipline and commitment along with both physical and mental toughness. These are all attributes that must be learned and practiced.

Running on a treadmill is comfortable, efficient and safe. But, it is not psychologically easy. It is really quite difficult to run and maintain pace on a treadmill. This is due, in part, to the perception that you are not going anywhere. You do not have the psychological cues that you are making progress, such as the wind in your face and the objects and scenery moving by. You also do not have other runners around you to keep you motivated.

Since running on the treadmill is usually a solitary activity, it helps build self-motivation and commitment. Running and maintaining your pace on the treadmill builds a mental "toughness" that will help you in your races and outside training runs.

Great For Beginners

The treadmill is ideal for beginning runners. Many new runners feel a bit intimidated by the sport and by more experienced runners. There is no reason for them to feel this way, but many do none the less. The treadmill gives these beginners a great place to start and to gain confidence in themselves so that feeling of intimidation melts away.

Most new runners start with walking. The treadmill is a great tool for incorporating those first running steps into a training program. It is very easy to add in very short surges of running. The treadmill provides them with a stable, level and dry surface in which to practice those first running steps.

The information provided by the display, such as time, speed, calories burned and distance traveled are all great motivational tools for beginners.

Heart Rate Training

Training by heart rate is a currently popular method of monitoring running intensity. Many mid and top level treadmills have built in heart rate monitoring capabilities. Some monitor heart rate by the use of a belt that wraps around your chest and others use monitoring pads on the treadmill handle grips.

A very useful function incorporated into some high end treadmills, is a program that regulates the treadmill speed and incline according to your heart rate. You simply tell the treadmill what your target heart rate range is. If your heart rate drops below your target range, the treadmill either speeds up or increases it's incline. If you rise above your target heart rate, the treadmill decreases it's speed or it's incline.

This is an essential feature for those that are running to rehabilitate after an illness, surgery or injury. Doctors often prescribe exercise performed at a specific heart rate. Heart rate feedback will keep these individuals exercising at the proper intensity.

Workout Variety

Treadmill workouts have an unlimited number of possible combinations of speed, distance and incline. You are able to design a run that will provide you with the exact workout that you desire. There is no outside training area that can give you everything you want in a workout. Only the treadmill gives you this kind of flexibility. This is an advantage to runners of all abilities, from a beginner to an elite runner.

Running Feedback

The console of today's treadmills give you a wealth of information. They tell you the distance you traveled, speed, average speed, calories burned, heart rate, pace and incline. This feedback provides you with important training information, training records and is also a motivational tool.

Air Pollution

Running outdoors in an area of high air pollution can be hazardous. Air pollution can come from automobile traffic, industrial exhaust, wood or coal burning or even forest fires. You should avoid running outside during times of high air pollution, especially if you suffer from asthma or any other respiratory problem. Running indoors on the treadmill is the ideal answer when you encounter these types of conditions.

Cons

The treadmill provides many benefits. But, as with everything, it is not perfect. Along with its many advantages, the treadmill does have some disadvantages.

Specificity

One of the "laws" of training, is the law of specificity. This simply means that your training should be as specific as possible to your training goal. In other words, your training should match your goal as closely as possible. You are training to run outside on the road, trail or track and run races, not to run on a treadmill.

Treadmill training has been proven, in scientific studies, to have very similar physiological effects, to outside or free-range running. In simpler terms, treadmill training gives you very similar training benefits when compared to free-range running. However, even though the physiological effects are very similar, it is not specifically the same as running outside. There are physical differences, which include lack of wind resistance, lack of changing terrain, running on a moving belt, bio-mechanical differences and psychological differences.

Lack of Wind Resistance

When running on the treadmill, you are obviously running in place. You are not running through the air. When you run outside you are running through the molecules of the air, which create resistance. The faster you run, the more of an effect the air resistance has on you. Studies have estimated that air resistance creates an increase in your running workload of between 2% and 10%, depending upon your running speed. The faster you run, the more of an effect the wind resistance has. You can compensate for the wind resistance by elevating the treadmill, one or two percent.

I suggest that you always elevate the treadmill 1 percent. That will make the effort level equal to running outside on flat ground.

Running Bio-Mechanics

In addition to the wind resistance problem, there is some evidence that running bio-mechanics are different when running on the treadmill. There have been very few conclusive studies done on the running form differences between treadmill and free range running. The studies that have been done have presented some rather conflicting data. Here is a brief summary of the reported running mechanics problems that have been associated with treadmill running.

• **Stride Length** - There have been reports of stride length being both longer and shorter than outside running. One study on the effects of treadmill running came up with some very interesting data. The study used one group of subjects that were very experienced runners and compared them to a group of new runners. The results showed that the more experienced group had longer strides when running on the treadmill, compared to their same pace when running outside. The interesting part is that the inexperienced group had the exact opposite result. They had shorter stride lengths on the treadmill than they did when running outside. More research is needed to determine why this happens and if it happens consistently to a large group of runners.

• **Longer Support Time** - Support time is the amount of time that your support leg spends on the ground. Some runners tend to spend more time on their support leg when running on the treadmill. In order to maximize your running efficiency your support time should be kept at a minimum. If your support leg is on the ground longer, you are probably not running as efficiently as you could be. This increase in support time is probably caused by an unconscious desire to provide a more stable running base on the moving and somewhat unstable treadmill.

• **Less Forward Lean** - Some studies have determined that some athletes run with less of a forward lean when running on the treadmill. This can cause more energy being wasted on up and down motion and less energy focused on forward momentum.

Running Surface

The even and soft surface of the treadmill is an advantage in many ways, but it does present one major disadvantage. When running outside you encounter uneven surfaces, stones, soft areas, hard areas, dry areas, wet areas and various combinations of these surfaces. The challenge of running over these surfaces improves your propreoception or the ability of your neuromuscular system to correct for the effect these types of surfaces have on your muscles and the position of your body parts and joints. This is critical to runners because it affects balance, power and running economy. Running on the treadmill removes this very important part of training.

Psychological Differences

Psychology plays a large role in the performance of runners. Treadmill running has several psychological factors that can affect the benefits of treadmill training.

• **Lack of Visual Cues** - When running outside you are moving past trees, buildings, automobiles and other people. When you are on the treadmill, you are not moving so you do not have those visual cues that signify movement. This can be very disconcerting and can lead to problems with running mechanics, confidence and training adherence.

• **Perception of Limited Room** - A properly fitted treadmill gives you more that sufficient room for even the longest running strides. However, the limited size of the running surface of the treadmill can give the impression that you may either "run off" the front of the machine or "fall off" the back. This commonly leads to a shortened and/or more vertical stride.

• **Lack of Confidence** - Many runners, especially more experienced runners that have been training most of their lives on the open road, do not trust the training benefits of treadmill running. This can be a self full filling prophecy. If you do not believe in something, it can and probably will have a negative effect on its benefits.

• **Boredom** - This is the daddy of all mental hurdles of treadmill training. Running in place can be boring and tedious. But take heart. This one is easily overcome

Availability of Gym Treadmills

If you do not own a treadmill and choose to use one at a gym, there is the problem of availability. Treadmills are very popular in a gym and it can be hard to find one not in use. When you do find one, there is usually a time limit of around 30 minutes per person, so you will not be able to do long workouts. The best way to solve this is to go to the gym during off hours. If there is no one waiting in line to use the treadmill, you can usually stay on the machine as long as you want.

Accuracy

As I mentioned earlier, the workouts on a treadmill can be more precise than outside running, because you can monitor exactly how fast and how far you are running. But, that is assuming that your treadmill is calibrated accurately.

Treadmills are notorious for being delivered from the factory with poor calibration. Most treadmill manufactures do not pay a lot of attention to exact accuracy. They do not believe that most users will notice the inaccuracy and many do not care. So, they do not put a lot of their resources into insuring accuracy.

It does not take much of an error to make a big difference in your training. An error of just 10% is disastrous. A 7:00 pace on the treadmill, could actually be a 7:40 pace. An error of this size can totally change the result and quality of your training run.

A good technician can calibrate your treadmill for you and it is well worth the money. If you just bought a treadmill, have it checked. The manufacturer warranty will cover the cost of calibration of any high quality treadmill.

Cost

Quality treadmills are not cheap. You can buy lower end treadmills at a discount store for $500 or less. But, this type of treadmill will not stand up to the abuse that a runner puts on it. It will also not operate smoothly, will not be as accurate, will be noisier and just not be an enjoyable experience.

A quality treadmill will start at around $1000 and go up to over $8000 for a club quality machine. This is a lot of money, but if you are going to use your treadmill on a consistent basis, it will be worth the extra cost to get a quality machine. You can usually find a good used treadmill in the classified ads. A good time to buy is in the several months after the New Year. Many people buy treadmills as a New Years resolution. They use them one or two times and then give up. You can usually pick one up for a bargain price. Also check with fitness specialty retail stores. Some of these shops will take used treadmills as trade ins or may have a treadmill returned by dissatisfied buyer. These machines can be purchased at discount prices.

This chapter is adapted from "Treadmill Training for Runners." For more information on this book go to www.runningplanet.com

Index

Printed in the United States
134239LV00004B/3/A